Women Rock Science

Megan A. Moreno
Rachel Katzenellenbogen

Women Rock Science

A Pocket Guide for Success in Clinical Academic Research Careers

Second Edition

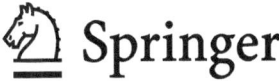 Springer

Megan A. Moreno
Pediatrics, Educational
Psychology
University of Wisconsin-
Madison
Madison, WI, USA

Rachel Katzenellenbogen
Pediatrics, Microbiology, and
Immunology
Indiana University School of
Medicine
Indianapolis, IN, USA

ISBN 978-3-031-48417-9   ISBN 978-3-031-48418-6   (eBook)
https://doi.org/10.1007/978-3-031-48418-6

This Springer imprint is published by the registered company Springer
Nature Switzerland AG
The registered company address is: Gewerbestrasse 11, 6330 Cham, Switzerland

Paper in this product is recyclable

Preface: Second Edition

We, Megan and Rachel, are so happy that you picked up this book! Five years have passed since we wrote the first edition of *Women Rock Science*, and we are excited to share this second edition with you.

The purpose of this book, and our motivation in writing it, remains the same. If you are a woman in clinically relevant science, we wrote this book for you. We are members of the same tribe, and we welcome you with open arms! In this second edition, we want to update some components of it to reflect the exciting diversity of who we all are as scientists.

First, we recognize that there are many populations of people who are underrepresented in medicine and clinically relevant sciences. So, we have added in content and reflections on the value of diversity in an individual's work and identity. Diversity, equity, and inclusion are key to excellence—and we have emphasized this in our second edition.

Second, we wanted to expand the focus of our book to acknowledge gender as a spectrum. We celebrate that there are other genders in science, and recognize that they too face challenges from not being the majority group. With that, we have added language inclusive of trans- and non-binary people, using both she/her pronouns and they/them pronouns. Additionally, our "**Women at Work**" sections are now called "**WOW! POW!**" to represent "Women at Work and People at Work." These speak to real-life situations of trans-, non-binary, and cis-women to highlight the importance of our peers in this field. Lastly, we brought in other women in leadership positions to speak about their experiences in our call-out section, "**Meaningful Moments.**" These are women who are high-level leaders in academics, and they are also members of communities that have been traditionally marginalized in science. Their thoughts and reflections on their paths are exciting to be able to include.

Third, we have expanded the leadership roles that we discussed in this edition. As women, we can rise to the top with our skillsets as scientists. The addition of other leadership positions, such as department chairs, are places we can lead other people in their future careers.

Finally, we have worked to make this second edition visually appealing by adding icons, diagrams, and visual aids to emphasize our points.

We are proud of the team effort that has made this book come to fruition!

Preface

If you are a woman (cis or trans) or non-binary person in clinically relevant science, we wrote this book for you. This includes MDs and DOs, such as physician-scientists, or physician educators doing research alongside teaching and clinical work. This includes PhDs or master's level scientists, doing work that will improve people's health and our understanding of disease. You may be a bench scientist, health services researcher, or medical education research fanatic. You may do research in lab coats, scrubs, jeans, or tutus (just kidding on the tutus, though that would be cool). You may have large teams backing you up or fly solo in most of your work. In all of these cases, we wrote this book for you. This book centers on ways to think about rocking your science and being part of the larger community of women and gender diverse scientists.

We had a few motivations in writing this book. One motivation was when reading other texts that provided strategies and advice about scientific careers, we noticed the pronouns were typically male. The case studies were usually focused on male scientists…unless of the case described a women scientist struggling to balance career and child-rearing. Another motivation for this book was the tremendous growth in the scientific and business literature on women and leadership. There are data that illustrate particular strategies for leadership and organization centered in areas that many women already have as strengths. We wanted a book with pronouns other than "he." We wanted to write a book that honored the unique strategies that women and gender diverse people can use in contributing to science. However, our goal was **not** to exclude those who do not identify as female. If you are reading this book and belong to another gender category, we are thrilled to have you along.

How to Use This Book

We suggest that it may be helpful to read, or skim, this book as a whole the first time through. The book is organized in a purposeful manner, as you will learn in Chap. 1. Chapter 1 establishes the framework of the book: the Socioecological Model. In that model, you as a scientist are in the middle, surrounded by your research team, then your institution, and then your professional societies. We explain the model and then nudge you to apply this framework and sketch out how it may apply to you and your science. We visit these themes in Chaps. 2–5 for early career faculty and then again in Chaps. 7–9 for the transition to the next stage of one's career. Each of these chapters provides information, evidence, and case studies of women scientists. Each chapter concludes with the opportunity to apply what you have learned to create sketches, lists, plans, or reflections that apply to your own science. Chapter 6 focuses on academic promotions, and the chapters that follow revisit key topics from the perspective of your mid to later career.

We welcome you to refer back to these chapters at different stages or when facing different experiences throughout your career. Chapter 6, focused on academic promotions, may be helpful to read when just starting a junior faculty position, so you know how to begin to build your promotion package successfully from the start. It then may also be helpful to revisit Chap. 6 yearly with your annual reviews and carefully read once more as your promotion process begins. Before going to your yearly academic conference, you may find it helpful to revisit Chap. 5 on national organizations and conferences. Even as you advance in your field and focus more on the topics in Chaps. 7–9, we invite you to re-read the earlier chapters as you become a mentor to early career scientists and want to center your advice and insights on their current issues.

How to Use Each Chapter

Each chapter begins with learning objectives to clarify the information we hope you will get from your reading. Throughout the chapter, we wanted to include a balance of evidence, advice, strategies, and voices from other women scientists. Therefore, you will note call-out sections in each chapter. One call-out is called "**Lessons from the Lab.**" This is a section in which we, as your authors and tour guides, share a little of our personal experiences. In another call-out section, "**Meaningful Moments**," we share pearls of wisdom, often from senior scientists in the field that we would consider role models. For each of these call-outs, we credit the scientist who was generous in sharing her reflections. We also highlight three "**Stories**" in this book from women whose career paths have been winding and fruitful. Finally, in the section "**WOW! POW!**" we share real-life situations of women and gender diverse scientists at work, with details changed to protect the innocent (and guilty). These sections are intended to highlight successful strategies and challenging situations.

Each chapter ends with **take-home points** we hope you will carry with you, as well as suggestions for **homework**. Yes, homework. Studies have shown that you learn more when you directly apply what you have learned, we wanted to provide some suggestions on direct application of content in each chapter. Some people may find it helpful to consider this true homework, while others may choose to think of it as extra credit.

At the end of the book, we include **references and resources**. There are many great resources out there, and we highlight ones linked to the content in and topic of each chapter.

Embrace Curiosity

We hope you will enjoy and benefit from this book, and it will spur you to continue to be curious about the process of rocking your science. We hope this curiosity will inspire you to continue to grow and learn your science, as well as continuing to pursue learning about the experience of being a woman or gender diverse scientist. We wrote this book inspired by our own curiosity. What we would learn? What could we share? And even, can we do this? And with this spirit of inquiry and curiosity, we share our first Meaningful Moments quote:

Meaningful Moments
The characteristic that has been the most powerful and sustaining in my career has been "curiosity." It has been the driver in both my clinical and research work. I like to understand and learn things about clinical conditions and understand or be able to explain (teach) as best as possible how things work together. For example, my interest in acute sinusitis in children stemmed from taking care of youngsters with orbital and central nervous system complications of sinusitis. Young children presenting with dramatic swelling and discoloration of the tissues surrounding the eye and teenage boys with fever, altered consciousness and focal neurologic signs were the stimulus to my interest. I wondered, what did sinusitis look like when it wasn't complicated? Some URIs become complicated by sinusitis but the majority don't. Why is that? How often do complications occur? Some cases of acute sinusitis resolve spontaneously, while others require treatment with antibiotics. Why is that and how can you tell?
    I sit in Grand Rounds every week and listen attentively.
    I am interested in almost every topic even though it may fall outside my realm of clinical care.
    I am curious.
    —Ellen Wald, MD

Stay in Touch

Writing this book started as a coffee conversation at a national meeting and grew over time to be a dream, and then a goal, and then an actual…thing. We hope it gives you strategies, new ideas, and a reminder of your own value. We also hope you will feel free to keep in touch; you can send us an email with feedback or your ideas on how best to rock science.

Madison, WI, USA   Megan A. Moreno
Indianapolis, IN, USA   Rachel Katzenellenbogen

Acknowledgments

We would be remiss if we did not thank the people who helped make this book, and its second edition, happen.

First to our reviewers and readers, whose input on the focus and scope of this book was invaluable: Jessica Babal, Kole Binger, Susan Ferguson, Amrutha Garimella, Aubrey Gower, Abby Hommer, Marina Jenkins, Pam Kling, Meisi Li, Caroline Mitchell, Tanya Mullins, HyunJu Park, Caroline Paul, Jenny Radesky, Ana Radovic, Christine Richards, Alan Schwartz, Kim Stevenson, Katie Sullivan, Nicholas Wallace, and FengHang Yao. Second, to our own mentors and colleagues who have supported and impressed us along the way: Steve Baylin, Aaron Carroll, Molly Carnes, William Chin, Dimitri Christakis, Bethany Deeds, Denise Galloway, Robert Golden, Ursula Kaiser, Steve Rosen, James Herman, Lia Vellardia, King Holmes, Fred Rivara, Larry Rosen, Beth Tarini, and Ellen Wald.

Finally, to our families. You inspire us to be better doctors and scientists and to lead by example for the next generation of academicians:

—Barney, Sydney, and Arthur

—Peter, Merritt, and Rin, and in memory of Fiona.

Thank you ~

Contents

Authors and Contributors

About the Authors

Megan A. Moreno, MD, MSEd, MPH is a professor of pediatrics and adjunct professor of educational psychology at the University of Wisconsin-Madison. She is principal investigator of the Social Media and Adolescent Health Research Team (SMAHRT); her research focuses on the intersection of technology and adolescent health. She has had continuous NIH funding since her initial K grant, as well as foundation, industry, and institutional support. She has authored over 180 research articles and was a lead author on the American Academy of Pediatrics (AAP) policy statement "Media Use Among School-aged Children and Adolescents."

In addition to research projects, SMAHRT also leads two research programs: (1) Technology and Adolescent Mental Wellness (TAM) program that has funded research, built a community of professionals around this topic, and includes a TAM Youth Advisory Board who are integral to the program's mission and function. (2) Summer Research Scholars program to provide adolescents exposure and experience in research in the area of adolescent health and social media as investigators.

She is a practicing adolescent medicine physician. Her leadership experience has included serving as division chief for General Pediatrics and Adolescent Medicine and Vice-Chair of Academic Affairs. She co-teaches a yearly graduate level course called Women in Leadership in Science, Health and Engineering: Gender Diversity in Leadership with Vice Provost Beth Meyerand (a contributor to this book). She is currently the interim chair of the Department of Pediatrics, and the co-medical director for the AAP's Center of Excellence on Social Media and Youth Mental Health with Dr. Jenny Radesky (a contributor to this book).

Rachel Katzenellenbogen, MD is the Richard E. and Pauline P. Klingler Professor of Pediatrics and a Professor of Microbiology and Immunology at Indiana University School of Medicine in Indianapolis. She conducts research on human papillomavirus (HPV) and how HPV initiates and drives cancer development and progression in people. She has had NIH funding since her initial K award, and she has conducted molecular biology research in the field of HPV domestically and internationally.

She has had a passion for mentoring researchers. While a faculty member at the University of Washington, she founded the Office for Teaching, Education and Research at the Seattle Children's Research Institute, and she co-taught Survival Skills for Scientific Research to graduate students. At Indiana University, she is a faculty member in the Morris Green Physician-Scientist Development Program in the Department of Pediatrics. She also is the program leader for the Indiana University Leadership Education in Adolescent Health (IU LEAH) training grant funded by HRSA.

She is chief of the Adolescent Medicine division, co-director of the Center for HPV Research at Indiana University, and co-leader of the Cancer Prevention and Control program at Indiana University Simon Comprehensive Cancer Center.

Contributors

Ruanne Barnabas, MBChB, DPhil is a graduate of the University of Cape Town, South Africa, where she received her medical degree. She received her research doctorate in medicine and clinical epidemiology from the University of Oxford, where she was a Rhodes Scholar. She completed residency in South Africa and her fellowship in Infectious Diseases at the University of Washington where she joined the faculty and was promoted to professor of Global Health and Medicine, and she currently is chief of Infectious Diseases at Massachusetts General Hospital (MGH).

Ruanne Barnabas' research has focused on interventions for HIV and STD treatment and prevention, and, more recently on COVID-19 prevention. She is particularly interested in novel approaches that increase access to services and has led clinical trials with companion health economic modeling to assess the potential impact of interventions as, for example, in the Delivery Optimization for Antiretroviral therapy (DO ART) Study, which evaluates the effectiveness and cost-effectiveness of decentralized, community-based ART initiation compared to clinic-based care. She also leads work assessing innovative strategies to increase access to care including lottery incentives and home delivery and monitoring of ART. She is the protocol chair of the KEN SHE Study to assess the impact of single-dose human papillomavirus (HPV) vaccination in Kenya. Recently, her work has extended to COVID-19 prevention within households. The ultimate aim of her work is to identify effective and scalable HIV, HPV, and infectious disease treatment and prevention strategies to increase access across diverse communities and promote equity in health. In addition to leading clinical trials and companion health economic modeling as an independently funded investigator, she also serves as an advisor to the World Health Organization and UNAIDS on cervical cancer elimination and treatment and prevention of HIV.

Shobhina G. Chheda, MD, MPH, FACP completed a combined internal medicine and pediatrics residency at Cornell University Medical College/North Shore University Hospital. She received her master's in public health at Saint Louis University School of Public Health. She joined the University of Wisconsin School of Medicine and Public Health faculty in 2001. A professor in the UW School of Medicine and Public

Health's Departments of Medicine and Pediatrics, she has been a leader in medical education locally and nationally.

In her role as associate dean for medical education, she has created, implemented, and now oversees our new medical student curriculum and assessment program. She was principal investigator on two consecutive educational grants from the Wisconsin Partnership Program: Re-envisioning Curriculum, Technology and New Programs Through a Health Equity Lens (2019–2022) and Building a Center for Innovation, Scholarship and Research in Undergraduate Medical Education (2023–2026) (CISR-UME). Nationally, she serves as chair of the Board of Directors for the Alliance of Academic Internal Medicine (AAIM), an organization representing over 11,000 physicians and administrative leaders committed to education and research in the field of internal medicine.

Rebecca Collins, PhD is a senior behavioral scientist at the RAND Corporation. Her research examines the determinants and consequences of health behavior. Current and recent projects focus on the effects of media on health. For the last decade, this work has focused on decreasing the vast discrepancy between the number of persons who need mental healthcare and the number who get it, through evaluation of publicly funded social marketing campaigns in California. Other work tested the influence of alcohol advertising on youth drinking and linked exposure to some types of sexual content in the media to adolescent sexual behavior and health. She co-led a National Academy of Sciences panel examining the association between sexual content in media and child health and was a member of the American Psychological Association (APA) task force investigating the primarily media-based sexualization of young girls in the USA. Her work for the U.S. military focuses on sexual behavior and health. Her research directly informed U.S. policy preserving abortion access for military service members, Department of Defense efforts to increase access to effective contraception among servicewomen, and the repeal of the military's Don't Ask Don't Tell policy. Addressing racial, eth-nic, gender identity, and sexual orientation equity is a key component of Collins' research. She is a fellow of the Association for Psychological Science. She has a Ph.D. in social psychology from UCLA. She also chairs RAND's Institutional Review Board, the *Human Subjects Protection Committee*.

Maggie Cooper is the communications lead for the Social Media and Adolescent Health Research Team (SMAHRT) and a communications specialist in the University of Wisconsin Department of Pediatrics. She works alongside a communications team to bridge the gap between research and the public.

Mary Dankoski, PhD is Executive Associate Dean for Faculty Affairs, Professional Development and Diversity and Lester D. Bibler Professor of Family Medicine. Her scholarly interests include the advancement of women and underrepre-sented faculty, the study of faculty vitality, how policies shape faculty life, and organizational and faculty development in academic medicine. From 2007 to 2012, she directed IUSM programs for the advancement of women, which led to IUSM receiving the Organizational Leadership Award from the Association of American Medical Colleges Group on Women in Medicine and Science (2009). She has served as President of the Indiana Association for Marriage and Family Therapy and on the Executive Board of Directors of the American Association for Marriage and Family Therapy as the chair of the Council of Division Presidents. In addition, she has served on multiple committees of the Association of American Medical Colleges Group on Faculty Affairs and was most recently named the Associate Editor of the Faculty Affairs Collection in MedEdPortal: The Teaching and Learning Journal. She completed her bachelor's degree in psychology at the University of Michigan and earned her PhD in mar-riage and family therapy with a graduate minor in women's studies from Purdue University.

Denise Galloway, PhD received her PhD in molecular biol-
ogy at City University of New York and did her postdoctoral
training in virology at Cold Spring Harbor Laboratories. She
is the director of the Pathogen Associated Malignancies
Integrated Research Center and a professor in the Human
Biology and Public Health Sciences Division at the Fred
Hutchinson Cancer Center. She holds the Paul Stephanus
Memorial Endowed Chair. She also is an affiliate professor in
Microbiology and Pathology at the University of Washington.
She has led research in the basic biology and immunology of
Human Papillomavirus and Merkel Cell Polyomavirus infec-
tions and how those infections cause cancers for more than
30 years. Her work has been recognized with election to
Fellowship in the American Academy of Arts and Sciences
and the Academy of the American Association for Cancer
Research and a National Cancer Institute's Outstanding
Investigator Award.

Isabel Garlough-Shah is a graduate of the University of
Wisconsin-Madison, where she double majored in journalism
and mass communications and gender and women studies.
Her skills reside in strategic communication and media
research with an emphasis on graphic design and data
analysis.

Ursula Kaiser, MD is professor of medicine at Harvard
Medical School and is the chief of the Division of
Endocrinology, Diabetes and Hypertension. She received her
medical degree at the University of Toronto, and she trained
in internal medicine and endocrinology at St. Michael's,
Toronto General, and Mount Sinai Hospitals in Toronto, and
Brigham and Women's Hospital in Boston. Her research
interests are in the biology of reproductive endocrinology
and how that is disrupted in disorders of the neuroendocrine
system. She acknowledges the influence of her research mentor, Dr. William Chin, whose support of women in science is
evidenced by the many women who trained in his laboratory
and have gone on to hold leadership positions in science and

medicine. She also would like to recognize the impact of Women in Endocrinology, a grassroots organization which has had a major influence on her development and success through their professionalism and continued and steadfast support of women's careers in the field of endocrinology.

Michelle Kimple, PhD is a faculty member in the Department of Medicine, Division of Endocrinology, Diabetes and Metabolism, at the University of Wisconsin-Madison and co-director of the University of Wisconsin Comprehensive Diabetes Center Islet Core. She is also a Research Health Scientist at the William S. Middleton Memorial Veteran's Hospital. Her research is focused on identifying new therapeutic targets for the β-cell dysfunction of diabetes and she is heavily involved in the training of future researchers and physician-scientists. She is a member of numerous professional organizations and is currently the chair-elect of the American Society for Pharmacology and Experimental Therapeutics Division for Molecular Pharmacology Executive Committee. Among the many awards she has received are the Department of Medicine's Puestow Research Award, awarded to a junior member of the Medicine faculty who has made a significant research contribution toward advancing the field of medicine, and the Vilas Life Cycle Professorship from the UW-Madison Women in Science and Engineering Leadership Institute and Office of the Provost. Finally, she is a passionate advocate for the destigmatization of mental health disorders. She studies how the disclosure of mental health disorder diagnoses impact, and the quality of institutional support affect, the ability of faculty to stay in a advance upwards through their careers.

Terri Laguna, MD received her undergraduate degree in molecular and cellular biology from the University of New Mexico and her M.D. from the University of California, San Francisco. She completed her Pediatric Residency and Chief Residency at the University of Washington and Seattle Children's Hospital. She completed her Pediatric Pulmonology

Fellowship training and obtained a master's degree in clinical science at the University of Colorado. She is the Division Head of Pulmonary and Sleep Medicine at Seattle Children's Hospital. She has built her research career in early lung disease in cystic fibrosis (CF). Her NIH R01 and Cystic Fibrosis Foundation (CFF) grant-funded work focuses on early infections in the CF airway and the role of anaerobic communities in the development of lung disease. She is a national mentor for the CFF and serves on NIH and CFF grant review study sections. She has been recognized for her teaching efforts as an Outstanding Faculty Educator by pediatric residents five times. She is active in diversity, equity, and inclusion (DEI) initiatives locally, regionally, and nationally. She has been active in many professional societies including the American Thoracic Society where she has served as co-chair of the DEI Advisory Group, Chair of the Program Committee and is the current chair of the Assembly on Pediatrics. Mentorship and sponsorship have been key throughout Dr. Laguna's career. She has had supportive women faculty across disciplines (Dr. Chris Wendt, Division Head of Adult Pulmonary and Critical Care Medicine at the Minneapolis VA Hospital and Dr. Stephanie Davis, chair of pediatrics at UNC) who have played instrumental roles in her career. Now, as an underrepresented minority in medicine in leadership positions, she seeks to use her platforms to elevate those faculty and trainees seeking to build careers in academic medicine.

Marsha Lopez, PhD, MHS has been involved in the study of health and disease for more than 30 years, participating in various aspects of projects ranging from medical and behavioral pharmacology to women's health and disability issues to epidemiology and surveillance, offering expertise in hands-on laboratory work, grant writing, study design, data collection, data analysis, and outcomes evaluation. In 2006, after training and career stops at Georgetown University, the Johns Hopkins University School of Hygiene and Public Health, University of Maryland, and Walter Reed Army Medical Center, she landed at the National Institute on Drug Abuse, where she is currently the chief of the Epidemiology Research Branch in the Division of Epidemiology Services and Prevention Research. In recognition of the impact early support made on her career trajectory, particularly as a woman who did not always take the traditional STEM route, she is now able to provide some of that reinforcement from the other side. She is thankful for the few but powerful women whose collaboration, humility, and humor continue to make the journey worthwhile (esp. BDG, KE), and for the opportunity to model for her kids Marco and Gigi how women truly rock.

Beth Meyerand, PhD is the vice provost for faculty and staff affairs at the University of Wisconsin-Madison. She joined UW-Madison's faculty in the Department of Medical Physics in 1998. A native of Rhode Island and a veteran of the United States Coast Guard, she values the privilege of service to others. She served as the first female chair in the Department of Biomedical Engineering and received the Slesinger Award for excellence in mentoring. She is honored to have chaired and served on the University Committee and the Divisional Committee for the Biological Sciences.

In her field of medical imaging, she is a fellow in the American Institute for Medical and Biological Engineering and the International Society for Magnetic Resonance in Medicine. She earned her B.S. degree in molecular biophysics and biochemistry from Yale University, a M.S. in biomedical engineering from the University of North Carolina at Chapel Hill, and a Ph.D. degree in biophysics from the Medical College of Wisconsin in Milwaukee. she has directed the graduate programs in the Departments of Medical Physics and Biomedical Engineering and serves as director of the Science and Medicine Graduate Research Scholars program, the largest program for graduate students of color on the UW-Madison campus.

Cary Moody, PhD is an associate professor of microbiology and immunology at the University of North Carolina at Chapel Hill. She studies the biology of human papillomavirus and how viral infection drives cancer development and progression. She received her PhD from Louisiana State University Health Sciences Center in Shreveport, and her postdoctoral training was in virology at Northwestern University.

Jenny Radesky, MD is an associate professor of pediatrics and director of the Division of Developmental Behavioral Pediatrics at the University of Michigan Medical School. She is a developmental behavioral pediatrician whose research focuses on family digital media use, child social-emotional development, and parent–child interaction. She uses a combination of observational, qualitative, and passive sensing methods to examine how parents and young children use mobile media throughout daily routines. She authored the 2016 American Academy of Pediatrics (AAP) digital media guidelines for young children and 2020 AAP policy on digital advertising to children. She is currently the chair of the AAP Council on Communications and Media.

Yolanda (Linda) Reid-Chassiakos, MD is a fellow of the American Academy of Pediatrics (AAP) and a fellow of the American College of Physicians. She served as a clinical assistant professor of pediatrics at the David Geffen School of Medicine, UCLA, from 1986 to 2021. After graduating from and completing her residency in pediatrics at the Georgetown University School of Medicine, she served as an awarded Lieutenant Commander in the US Navy, as the Assistant Head of the Ambulatory Branch of Pediatrics at the Naval Hospital, Bethesda, and as an assistant professor of pediatrics at the Uniformed Services University of the Health Sciences. After her honorable discharge, she joined the Department of Health and Human Services' Office of Disease Prevention and Health Promotion and served as a medical editor and feature reporter for the evening Eyewitness news at the CBS affiliate in Washington, DC. She then moved to Lifetime Medical Television in Los Angeles as a medical editor, writer, and host of national and international educational programming for healthcare professionals and the public and developed and hosted programs and features for media such as the NBC Network *Sex, Drugs, and Rock 'n Roll*, Lorimar-Telepictures, and You TV. During her 13-year tenure as an associate physician diplomate at UCLA's Arthur Ashe Health Center, she also served as a staff writer for the television series, Family Medical Center. She became the executive director and chief medical officer of the Klotz Student Health Center at California State University, Northridge, serving CSUN for 21 years (including as campus pandemic manager) until her retirement in December 2021. Her features and essays have been published in the *Washington Post, Baltimore Sun, Woman's Day*, *Salon.com*, the *Los Angeles Times*, the *Los Angeles Daily News*, *HuffPost*, and *Tribune International*. She is a member of the Council on Communications and Media of the American Academy of Pediatrics and served on its Executive Committee for 6 years. She was the lead author of the AAP Technical Report "Children, Adolescents, and Digital Media" (2016) and co-author of "Digital Advertising to Children" (2020).

She would like to acknowledge for their collaboration and mentorship her AAP colleagues Dr. Megan Moreno, Dr. Jenny Radesky, Dr. Dimitri Christakis, Dr. Corinn Cross, Dr. David Hill, Dr. Nusheen Ameenudin, and Dr. Vic Strasburger as well as Dr. Deborah Shlian, MD, MBA, editor of Lessons Learned: Stories from Women Physician Leaders and Lessons Learned: Stories from Women Leaders in STEM.

Stephanie Craig Rushing, PhD, MPH is a Principal Investigator at the Northwest Portland Area Indian Health Board. Her work has focused on designing and evaluating multimedia programs to improve American Indian/Alaskan Native adolescent health using mixed methods community-based participatory research strategies. She completed her Masters of Public Health at Boston University and her PhD in Public Administration and Policy at Portland State University.

Maria Trent, MD, MPH   is a professor of Pediatrics, American Health, and Nursing at Johns Hopkins University, director of the Division of Adolescent/Young Adult Medicine, and the senior associate dean of Diversity and Inclusive Excellence at the Johns Hopkins University School of Medicine. She is a Bloomberg Endowed professor of American Health and an independent research scientist. As such, she is the principal or key investigator on multiple research projects and training grants funded by the National Institutes of Health (NIH) and other funding agencies in domestic and international arenas. A significant focus of Dr. Trent's research and clinical interest has been on reducing adolescent and young adult sexual and reproductive health disparities, with particular attention to sexually transmitted infections and HIV prevention and intervention. She is a past president of the Society for Adolescent Health and served two terms as chair of the Executive Committee for the Section on Adolescent Health within the American Academy of Pediatrics. She is a sought-after speaker and the author of scientific research articles and other forms of health publications, including serving as lead author of the landmark American Academy of Pediatrics policy statement, "The Impact of Racism on Child and Adolescent Health," and co-editor of a forthcoming text *Untangling the Threads of Racism: A Primer for Pediatric Health Professionals (AAP Publishing)*. Professional organizations and the lay press have recognized Dr. Trent for her work, and she has emerged as an important voice and forceful advocate for the health and well-being of young people and those who care for them.

Heidi Wagner, OD, MPH   received her Doctor of Optometry degree from the Ohio State University and her Master of Public Health degree from the University of Massachusetts at Amherst. She is a Professor of Clinical Optometry at the Ohio State University where she serves as the director of Extern Programs. Previously, she was a professor of optometry at Nova Southeastern University where she served the College as Department Chair from 2001 to 2011. She is a diplomate in the Cornea, Contact Lenses and Refractive Technologies Section of the American Academy of Optometry as well as a distinguished practitioner and fellow in the National Academies of Practice. She was the principal investigator for the Nova Southeastern University CLEK (Collaborative Longitudinal Evaluation of Keratoconus) Clinic, a multicenter observational study funded by the National Eye Institute. She currently serves as co-chair of the Contact Lens Assessment in Youth (CLAY) study group. She would like to do a shout out to her dean and mentor, Karla Zadnik.

Ellen Wald, MD is the Alfred Dorrance Daniels Professor on Diseases of Children in the Division of Infectious Disease and was the Chair of Pediatrics at the University of Wisconsin-Madison. She earned her medical degree from SUNY Downstate Medical Center in Brooklyn, New York. She completed her residency in pediatrics at Kings County Hospital in Brooklyn and her fellowship in infectious disease at the University of Maryland Hospital in Baltimore.

In 1997, she received the Pediatrician of the Year award from the Pennsylvania Chapter of the American Academy of Pediatrics, and in 2001 she was honored with the Howard Mermelstein Award for Excellence in Pediatrics. She received an Alumni Achievement Award in 2018 from SUNY Downstate Medical Center for her significant contributions to the medical profession. She has been recognized for her teaching ability on many occasions, including in 2001, when she received the Resident Teaching Award at the Children's Hospital of Pittsburgh and in 2008 when she was the recipient of a clinical teaching award from the pediatric housestaff at the University of Wisconsin. She served as chair of the Department of Pediatrics at the University of Wisconsin-Madison School of Medicine and Public Health from 2006 to 2022.

She would like to recognize Jane Pitt. "I met Jane when I was a PL3 which was also the year that I served as chief resident. She was a young scientist who had recently completed her training at Columbia University, and she came to my residency to join the Division of Infectious Disease. She seemed very self-assured and knowledgeable and was an excellent teacher. Jane was the only faculty member who ever invited me to her home with a small group of other residents. She was the first person I ever heard use the word 'aminoglycoside' to describe a class of antimicrobials to which gentamicin and kanamycin belonged and provide a framework in which to consider the appropriate use of antibiotics. She was my inspiration to pursue Infectious Diseases as a specialty. I can't say that she mentored me but did serve as a role model."

Garrett Waterman is a communications specialist at SMAHRT. He majored in communications and rhetorical science with a focus on health communication at the University of Wisconsin-Madison. He has managed multimedia campaigns strategies for new publications, conferences, and youth programs. His skills encompass video editing, graphic design, long form writing, and social media curation.

Susanne Wells, PhD is a professor of pediatrics and the director of the Epithelial Carcinogenesis and Stem Cell Program. She received her PhD in molecular genetics at the State University of Stony Brook and her postdoctoral training was in molecular virology at Harvard Medical School. She studies the biology of squamous cell cancer development and progression due to infection and non-infection related causes.

Jennifer Whitehill, PhD is an associate professor of Health Policy and Management. She is the graduate program director in the Department of Health Promotion and Policy. Her research centers on preventing injuries, from a variety of mechanisms (e.g. motor vehicle crashes, poisonings, gun violence), among youth and young adults. Her current work focuses on substance use as a risk factor for injury and on the injury implications of cannabis legalization. She also studies the role of new media technologies such as mobile devices and social networking sites as both a risk factor for injury and a possible avenue for prevention.

Chapter 1
The Framework for This Book: The Socioecological Model

In this chapter we will introduce the main framework for this book: the socioecological model, and how it is useful to think about and plan your career.

If you are a junior scientist, you have undoubtedly experienced focus on you as an *individual*. You have been asked to define your individual interests, skills, and strengths. You develop a personal research mission and individual mission statement. Your accomplishments have been assessed at an individual level, and much of your work writing proposals or manuscripts likely felt pretty solo. If you are a mid-level or more senior scientist, you may have experienced these processes as well as the opportunity to self-reflect or redefine yourself and your research interests. Regardless of your stage of career, you cannot rock your science alone. Really. And why would you want to? Science, like many other grand adventures, is best pursued with others at your side. Hermione worked alongside Harry and Ron. T'Challa leaned on Shuri in tough times. Katniss partnered with Peeta and Haymitch.

As you consider your own grand career adventure, we invite you to reflect on your *context*, or the people, resources, and structures that surround you as an individual. Your context may include the mentors who provide feedback on your proposals, the colleagues who you meet for coffee, and the

M. A. Moreno, R. Katzenellenbogen, *Women Rock Science*, https://doi.org/10.1007/978-3-031-48418-6_1

role models you strive to emulate within your institution. Your context may include your Institutional Review Board chair who gives you helpful feedback, your black, indigenous and people of color (BIPOC) affinity group who provides you a supportive space, the administrative assistant who exactingly double-checks your manuscripts, and your clinic scheduler who always wants to add on an extra patient for you to see. Your context presents both opportunities and challenges to you every day. Without your context, little would get done in your day-to-day. However, context is more than that, as it represents your unique position within a larger society of faculty at your institution, and scientists within your field.

Further, reflect for a moment on the long game of your career, which will include your successes and failures, your development as a scientist and your pathway through a research career. In this chapter we hope it will become clear that understanding and integrating your context into your work and life is essential to long-term productivity, growth, and happiness. We will use the socioecological model to guide the approach to considering your research context and use this approach to guide the framework by which we present information to you within this book.

For this chapter, we will first define and explore the socio-ecological model, and the ways in which this framework can be integrated into your path, your career, and your area of research. We will then review two additional key frameworks to keep in mind as you navigate this book: mentorship and leadership. We will discuss how these frameworks can be integrated into your overall context.

The Socioecological Model

The socioecological model (SEM) is a theory-based framework for understanding the interactive effects of personal and environmental factors that determine behaviors. A typical socioecological model is drawn as a series of concentric circles, with the individual at the center, followed by levels including interpersonal, community, organizational, and policy/enabling environment.

The SEM has been used in a variety of ways for project design as well as research. It has been applied to explain violence in a community, to improve healthy eating in schools, and to design a colorectal cancer screening program. The telescoping framework of the SEM is useful in thinking from small to large, from individual to society, and from local to global.

To be a successful and satisfied scientist, making connections and using resources across these contexts is critical. Figure 1.1 shows the application of the SEM to this book, and how we will approach the information within this book, linking you to and across your contexts.

The individual will be the focus of Chap. 2. It is probably obvious, but you are the scientist here. You are the source of your greatest ideas and best plans. Wherever you are at your stage of the grand adventure that is your career right now, you got yourself there. And to succeed and thrive, you need to give yourself the time and resources to engage in ongoing reflection and learning.

The level closest to the individual is typically *the interpersonal context*, which for an academic clinician researcher should include close colleagues and mentors. This *interpersonal context* level also includes your immediate research group, which includes your research staff, interns and students who work for and with you. In this book we will refer to this group as *your research team*. This *interpersonal context* may include those who are important to you in your personal life as well, such as your family and friends. Those individuals who you consider in this level of the SEM are your strongest and closest sources of support, people with whom you can be yourself, share your frustrations or failures, and celebrate your successes. They can lift you up when you are down and cheer you on as your work receives recognition. Maintenance of these relationships is critical at every stage of your career,

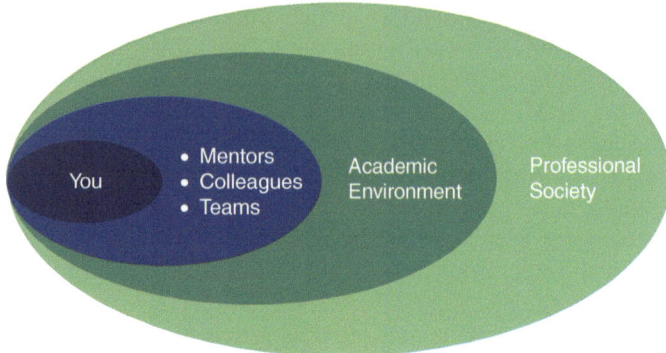

FIGURE 1.1 The socioecological model

and we will focus on your research team, colleagues, and mentors in Chap. 3.

In the academic world, your next level in the SEM is typically your *academic environment*, represented by your institution or university. This environment includes:

- Colleagues *within* your division and department
- Colleagues *across* different disciplines around your university
- Organizations such as the Institutional Review Board, Animal Care and Environmental Health
- Groups supporting key aspects of your identity such as lesbian, gay, bisexual, transgender, queer/questioning, intersex (LGBTQI+), BIPOC, ongoing conditions or disability, or areas of academic interest
- Resources such as libraries, core facilities, seminars, and collaborative space and
- Academic staff whose job includes providing support for your promotion, grant submissions, and managing meetings

Knowing your institution means you may have access to campus grants, training programs, or sources of (and for) mentees. Further, knowing your institution and developing relationships across campus can contribute to your success and feeling of engagement in your place of work. Your academic environment will be the focus of Chap. 4.

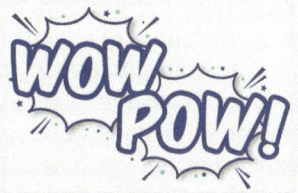

As a reminder, throughout this book we will use call-out boxes to illustrate examples of women at work (WOW) and people at work (POW) and how they represent the topics discussed in that chapter.

Khira is a gastroenterology fellow whose area of interest is in the effects of obesity on the liver, and her most recent study examined MRI changes noted in the liver among women with obesity. Her interpersonal context includes her research mentor who is a Professor of Radiology, her clinical mentor in the Division of Gastroenterology, her co-fellows, as well as her spouse. She is also active in her institution's LGBTQI+ community. Her fellowship is in an academic medical center within a private university; that represents her institutional context. Because her work crosses disciplinary lines, she spends time in professional societies focused on gastroenterology as well as professional societies focused on obesity. Through clearly defining these roles for herself, she was able to integrate her SEM vision into her application for a career development grant, as well as make the case for additional conference time to attend national meetings for both gastroenterology and obesity. While attending her first GI conference, she was able to quickly find supportive colleagues through attending the LGBTQI+ trainee dinner.

The furthest level out from the center in the SEM is your larger *professional society*. For some scientists, you may have more than one professional society to represent distinct aspects of your work. For example, many pediatrician researchers belong to the American Academy of Pediatrics, a large organization contributing to pediatric education, advocacy, and policy. Pediatrician researchers may also belong to the Society for Pediatric Research or the American Pediatric Society, each a large professional group representing all types of pediatric research. Further, pediatric subspecialists may also belong to their subspecialty organization, be that adolescent medicine, cardiology, or neonatology. Navigating your relationships within these organizations, and seeking opportunities to contribute within larger institutions, can increase the impact of your work and your career opportunities. It will be the focus of Chap. 5.

The good news is that most academic clinicians are already prepared to think about navigating different contexts. The "typical" academic professional's work includes all three aspects of what has been called the "*academic 3-legged stool*." The three legs of this stool include clinical work or service for non-clinicians, teaching, and research. Figure 1.2 illustrates this framework, and how these areas of work can overlap and enhance each other. For example, if you study obesity interventions, it is wise to develop and nurture your teaching on topics related to obesity. This may include delivering a medical student lecture on obesity prevention and intervention, or a talk in the nursing school on obesity 101, or speaking in a seminar about behavioral health related to nutrition or physical activity. Seeking opportunities for integration of your area of research and teaching into your clinical world both further cements your skills and allows for continuous exposure to your study population and their experiences. These clinical experiences can provide endless opportunities to develop new research ideas. Not everyone can achieve perfect alignment of their research, education, and clinical work, but seek-

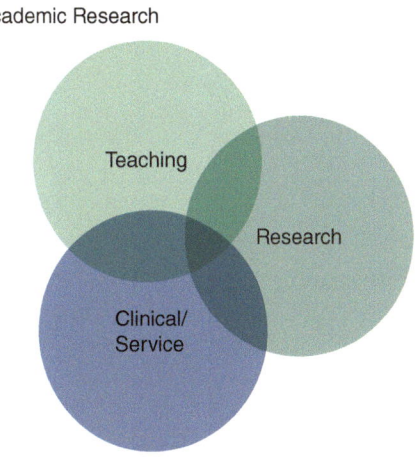

Academic Research

FIGURE 1.2 The "3-legged stool" of academic medicine

ing opportunities to integrate your key areas of interest is an important strategy to make your work count in every area of your effort.

A final application of the SEM to your research is to consider your area of research focus as its own SEM. Considering the grand scheme of everything that could be a research focus in your topic area, your own area of research is likely to be narrow. By definition, that is the path to success, to go deeply into a specific research topic and question and, through that, make a difference. For example, a successful researcher may study drug resistance in tuberculosis, but not every aspect of its prevention, diagnosis, risk factors, and novel drug discovery. Thus, your own research focus will fit into a larger body of scientific work. This is not meant to diminish your work; it is meant to put your research in the larger context of the world of science. Identifying your research interests, and your specific approach to those interests, is the focus of Chap. 2.

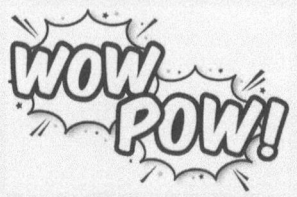

Cristina is pursuing a PhD in communication arts; her work focuses on how patients choose to communicate about serious illnesses such as cancer. She has developed a niche within the Communication field in this area. She sees her work within the larger body of work on patient communication styles, with some overlap in the area of physician-patient communication. She has also developed a growing reputation within the field of cancer research, and she is frequently sought out as a conference speaker on this topic. She sees her primary niche in health communication, within the larger context of the field of communication. Since her work contributes to cancer research, she sees her "general scientific research" area as intersecting with cancer research.

Figure 1.3 shows this relationship, demonstrating your area of research focus within a niche of research. Over your career, you may indeed develop from a narrow focus to a niche in which you pursue related studies in a given area. Working with collaborators can also expand your area of focus into a niche. Your body of work will lead to advancements in general scientific research and knowledge, and that will push biomedical sciences forward in understanding and clinical care.

FIGURE 1.3 A researcher's
socioecological model

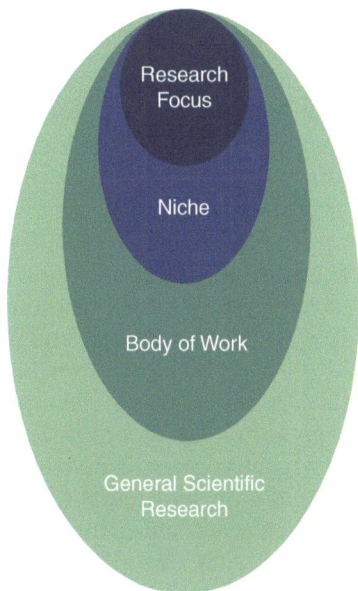

Mentorship: It Takes a Village (or a SEM)

Mentorship is critical to a career in science. There is little chance of success in a research career without having a mentor and becoming a mentor. Mentors provide teaching in research skills such as planning a project, managing staff, and writing papers. Mentors also provide role modeling; we watch them to understand how to react in a given situation. Mentors provide us feedback on where we are and what we are doing. Mentors also provide support; when the going gets rough we can turn to mentors for guidance, reassurance, or redirection.

Research on mentoring suggests that mentoring contributes to an individual's career development in the areas of research, career satisfaction, and perceived institutional support. The mentoring process provides a means by which junior faculty can develop professional academic skills including career management, knowledge about academic medicine, and networking. Thus, mentorship can assist you in navigating the SEM and expanding your reach outward to your institution and society.

However, mentorship is not automatic or guaranteed in an academic clinical career. A 2006 meta-analysis found that less than 50% of medical students and less than 20% of faculty had a mentor. Further, women perceived they had more difficulty getting mentors than men. The process of finding mentors takes time. You may note the plural was used in the previous sentence because every academic clinician scientist needs mentors to represent the distinct parts of a job, or different skillsets that are needed. Chapter 3 describes tips on navigating this process and the time it takes to find mentors. It is work, it is a process, and it is absolutely necessary.

As you build your own research team, you are likely to start to provide mentorship to others. These early mentorship experiences are important. Even if you do not feel "ready" to be a mentor, chances are you have remarkable things to offer. Studies have shown that the benefits of mentoring extend to both mentors and mentees. Being a mentor allows you to consider your own SEM and context, as well as your own place in other people's SEMs. In the long term, mentoring has been proposed as a solution to reduce burnout and enhance career satisfaction.

Meaningful Moments
I believe that the days of a solitary investigator, working in his/her laboratory in isolation, are long behind us. Science is now so sophisticated and complex, none of us can be expert in all things. It is much more efficient and more likely to lead to success to develop deeper expertise in one area and to work with collaborators who have complementary expertise, rather than trying to do it all by oneself. This approach will allow the investigator to move science forward more effectively and to be a lifelong learner, learning from collaborators. In fact, I believe that "collaboration versus independence" is not correct—there is not "either/or" in this statement—the two are complementary, not competing! One can be independent and yet collaborate.
—Ursula Kaiser, MD

Transformational Leadership: Women and Context

Research demonstrates good news on this front: working within a context is a skill that is typically strong within women. A meta-analysis representing 45 studies compared leadership skills between men and women. They were particularly interested in *transformational leadership*.

Transformational leaders are skilled in working within contexts to achieve results. They establish themselves as role models by gaining the trust of others. They are transparent about their future goals and develop plans to achieve those goals. They mentor and empower those they work with, clearly reaching across the different levels in the SEM into their communities, institutions, and societies.

Transformational leadership styles can also be understood in contrast to a more traditional leadership style of *transactional leadership*. Transactional leaders establish give-and-take relationships that appeal to the self-interest of those below them. In transactional leadership, people are expected to perform their duty, stay in their place, and be rewarded for completing their tasks.

A third type of leadership has been defined as *laissez-faire,* a sort of non-leadership that is distant and non-directive.

In general, most people have a more dominant style and integrate aspects of the other styles into their daily practice.

In previous research, women were more skilled at transformational leadership, particularly in the areas of giving support and encouragement to others. The good news is that transformational leadership is considered the most effective for leading the modern organization. Previous research also suggests that women's leadership approaches, using transformational styles, are typically more effective compared to transactional or laissez-faire.

A separate meta-analysis found that women are more likely to adopt a participative and collaborative style compared to men. The reason for this difference is not attributed to biology or genetics. It has been suggested that women are more likely to get better results when using these approaches compared to autocratic or dictatorial styles that are sometimes found to be jarring for women. Less is known about leadership styles for other genders, and studies in this area are needed. Anecdotal evidence supports that individuals who identify as transgender (trans) or non-binary may have more in common with women's leadership styles compared to men's, as they are also members of an underrepresented group in science.

Thus, in considering you as an individual in context, these findings suggest that women, trans- and non-binary scientists can be adept at leveraging relationships across contexts. This has benefits in job satisfaction; if your colleagues and team members appreciate and look up to you, you feel valued. This also has benefits in productivity; if your research team members feel connected to you, they are more likely to be invested in your work and your success. If you respect and promote your research team members' success, they are more likely to stay with you and that means less turnover in your lab….less money and time spent in onboarding, training, and adjusting your team's work when people come and go.

A final issue to recognize and address in considering gender is that traditional cis-gender schemas are present today, as they were a decade or a century ago. Gender schemas refer to implicit, or nonconsciousness, assumptions about sex differences. In many professions, including science, there is an assumption about men being superior compared to women. While strides have been made to eliminate these outdated stereotypes and gender schemas, they still exist. Further, women, non-binary, and trans people represent a growing minority in science, and this can leave them vulnerable to poor behavior by the majority. Stories and studies have illustrated that sexual harassment remains a significant issue in science. One of the many ways to overcome and address these schemas, and build a network you can turn to if you experience sexual harassment, is to build relationships across multiple layers of your SEM. This approach can connections for yourself and others and contributing to a new scientific society with women and gender diverse people as equal partners, contributors, and collaborators.

The Third Person for This Book

The first edition of this book was the first of its kind as a guide focusing on women in science in academic clinical and biomedical research. In our initial decision to write this book in 2015, we had the lofty and passion-driven goal of contributing to the development of women scientists' careers so that all of science includes women as equal partners, innovators, and leaders. Groups other than cis males have historically been underrepresented in science (alongside other minority groups). In preparing for this book, we read many other science guidebooks. Many of these books had excellent content and contributed to ideas shared in this book. However, we noted that most default pronouns were "he." We were also disappointed that example cases in these books usually focused on men with male mentors. We were a little miffed (to put it mildly) to discover that a common "example case" of a woman scientist involved stories of scientists who wanted to cut back on their work after having children. For the first edition of this book, we wanted to focus on advancing women in science and going beyond the male focus of existing guidebooks.

In this new edition, we recognize the importance of taking a broader lens of gender to include women, trans, and non-binary people. Rather than call-out boxes with "women at work" as in the first edition, we have updated this edition to label call-out boxes with WOW (women at work) and POW (people at work) to embrace inclusivity. While cis-women continue to be underrepresented in science, trans, non-binary, agender, and two-spirit scientists are as well. We need diversity in science to make science better. We need new voices to share the experiences of diverse scientists and inspire the next generation of scientists. We need the hes, shes, theys, and xes to be part of this work. Our focus in this book will be on scientists who identify as female and non-binary. In that spirit, when we use a third person pronoun, we will avoid the default pronoun of "he" and have chosen the default pronouns of "she" or "they."

Meaningful Moments
As an undergraduate student in Germany, I applied for an exchange program with the Department of Microbiology at SUNY Stony Brook. To this day I still don't know why. I had no intention of leaving Germany. But I also did not enjoy my biology major and needed a change. I was awarded a slot, went to the USA, and fell in love with the research environment that I experienced there.
—Susanne Wells, PhD

Take-Home Points

The SEM is a useful framework to consider your place as an academic clinician scientist within a larger framework.
   Mentorship is integral to your career and within the SEM.
   Leadership skills, particularly transformational leadership, also integrate context and can be a strength in women and gender diverse scientists.

Homework
- Draw a SEM representing your current context. Use black ink for your current SEM, and a distinct color of ink (sparkly purple? we will never tell) to add in places where you would like to enhance it.
- Draw a SEM representing your research context.
- Save these drawings to revisit during or after reading this book.

   Real-life SEM example (thank you Dr. Kimple!) (Fig. 1.4).

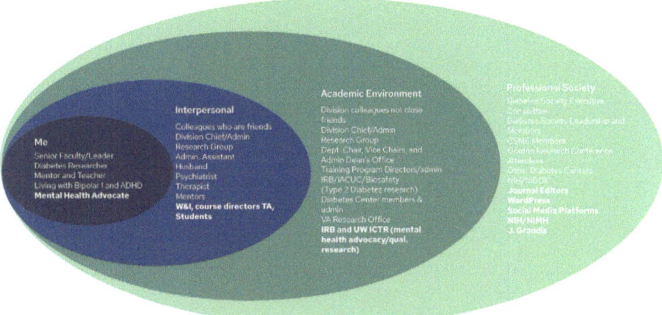

FIGURE 1.4 Dr. Michelle Kimple's example of a socioecological model. Note that the text in regular font represents current relationships, and the text in bold represents goals for future relationships

Chapter 2
You as a Scientist

In this chapter we will approach three broad topics: your passion, your values, and your work style. As described in Chap. 1, these topics are part of the innermost circle of the socioecological model, which is the individual (YOU, baby!). Each of these aspects of who you are is interlinked and affects your research career. Each requires you to focus on yourself to best understand what and how you want to lead your career as a scientist. In each section we will ask you to reflect and define what your passions, values, and work style are or will be. These are topics you will return to throughout your career, to reaffirm or strengthen, and to modify or redirect. Consistent periodic self-reflection will best allow you to move forward in your career and really rock science to its core.

Unique Strengths of Women Scientists

People have studied gender and leadership styles, and women have been consistently identified as more likely to have leadership styles that are collaborative. Women are commonly identified as leaders who elevate their team members, identify others' strengths and bring them out, and create a work environment in which people's voices are heard. This is all good news, as science can flourish when people feel sup-

© The Author(s), under exclusive license to Springer Nature Switzerland AG 2024
M. A. Moreno, R. Katzenellenbogen, *Women Rock Science*,
https://doi.org/10.1007/978-3-031-48418-6_2

ported to contribute their ideas. A supportive and open work environment in science is also important when things go wrong, as your research staff will be more willing to express concern about a project direction, or identify when something is going wrong, if they feel safe in doing so.

What Is Your Passion?

As a scientist, you are innately interested in the study of the unknown. You are inquisitive. You want to discover how and why things are the way they are. With that inquisitive nature comes a passion. However, how do you know what your passion is? As we train, we may find that *many* things are interesting. We like chemistry, biology, epidemiology, statistics, population health, and more. We enjoy social studies, anthropology, and history. That being said, as an independent researcher, each of us needs to take the time and think through what we are truly passionate about—passionate enough to not just learn about but to spend our careers focusing on, garnering answers to our questions. In order to determine your passion, you need to take the time to think.

Self-reflection is important. Consider:

- What do you enjoy thinking about?
- Asking about?
- Talking about?
- Working on? What ideas do you find yourself returning to at odd moments—walking your dog, cooking a meal, driving in a car?
- What topics do you talk about and have trouble *stopping* once you get started?
- What keeps you up at night?
- What do you dream about, and even find solutions to, in your dreams?

Through self-reflection you can identify what is important to you in research and what pushes you to engage fully. There are many ways to have this self-reflection. You can truly just set aside time to think about it, you can talk about it with other people, or you can get your thoughts on paper through writing. However, at least annually you should come back to review your passions and your previous thoughts and conclusions. To make this self-reflection happen, you will need to schedule it. Block an hour or two on your calendar, and dive in. Do not check email, do not multitask, do not overwrite your schedule for this. Prioritize this time to think, reflect, and understand what you are doing in your work and why. By doing this, you will see that your passions can deepen. You will also see that your passions can migrate over time. With this first self-reflection, and then pausing annually for re-evaluation, you will keep yourself in your best path to success in research.

Meaningful Moments

I suspect a thousand little nudges—from my family, teachers, peers, and life experiences—brought me to the field of public health and my current occupation.

In grade school my parents nurtured interest in experimentation and annual science fairs—elaborate, closely-monitored experiments involving trays of seedlings grown under different light conditions, homemade devises measuring the expansion and retraction of metals when heated and cooled, and microscopes to observe swabbed cheek cells. In elementary and middle school, I participated in Odyssey of the Mind, an international competition that blended problem solving, construction, engineering and mechanics, with art, language and theater. Each year, our seven-member team would be given a "challenge" in the fall, and would present our solution at local, state, and international competitions in the spring. Over years of competition, this small team taught me the value of creativity and thinking outside the box, and that complex problems take time and iteration to solve; that you won't necessarily get right it the first time, but must try different approaches and configurations to refine your solution. From a rather early age, this team of peers showed me the importance of teamwork and the value that each individual brings to collective efforts, and to surround yourself with peers who will push you to do your very best work. It was undoubtedly this experience and success that gave me the confidence to pursue the sciences in college, majoring in Biology with a Chemistry minor.

—Stephanie Craig Rushing, PhD, MPH

WHAT and WHY

As a part of self-reflection on research and your passions, you need to think about TOPICS (the WHAT). The TOPIC that you are passionate about is important to identify. The topic will affect the way you fund your research. Institutes and Centers at the National Institutes of Health (NIH) are structured around topic areas. For example, if you study breast cancer, your research programs would most likely be funded through the National Cancer Institute. Non-profit organizations that fund research are even more topic-based than federal agencies. The American Cancer Society may want to support your work if you propose a project on breast cancer; a foundation focused on autism would toss your application aside. The topic that you chose for your research will also affect your job. Your research topic must find a home within a department that conducts and supports work in that field. If you study T-cell immunology, you may choose to join an immunology department or another affiliated program. You would be a poor candidate in the epidemiology department. The topic that you study will also affect your collaborators. If you study drug use in adolescents, your collaboration with psychiatrists, neurologists, public health agencies, schools, epidemiologists, and statisticians will be critical. It is less likely that you will work with gerontologists. We are often interested in many things, but this exercise in self-reflection is to understand the singular topic that rises to the top among your passions. This may seem intuitively obvious, but determining the critical importance of your topic area within your passions cannot be overemphasized.

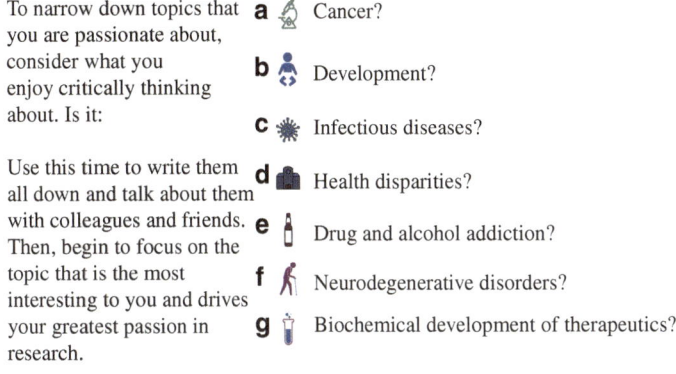

To narrow down topics that you are passionate about, consider what you enjoy critically thinking about. Is it:

a Cancer?

b Development?

c Infectious diseases?

Use this time to write them all down and talk about them with colleagues and friends. Then, begin to focus on the topic that is the most interesting to you and drives your greatest passion in research.

d Health disparities?

e Drug and alcohol addiction?

f Neurodegenerative disorders?

g Biochemical development of therapeutics?

(a–g) Representations of areas of research focus

Once you have identified the topic area of research about which you are most passionate, you next will need to determine WHY the topic that is compelling to you. WHY is key. Many people are fascinated and passionate about a topic, but they will want to answer questions about that topic for very different reasons. The answer is never just "because it is cool." It is also not because it is what you know and feel comfortable studying. There is a context behind your passion about a topic. That context is your WHY.

Let's say you are interested in studying attention deficit hyperactivity disorder. What intrigues you?

- It is the *clinical implications* of a disease or risk factor?
- The *biologic understanding* behind a disease or outcome?
- The *population outcomes* from a group at risk?
- The *policy implementation* to decrease risk, morbidity, and mortality?

Meaningful Moments

I did not intend to be a physician scientist. During my residency, I had no clue even what that meant! During my pediatric pulmonology fellowship, I found myself drawn to the cystic fibrosis (CF) population. I enjoyed getting to know the families and partnering with them over time. I soon found out what a devastating disease CF was, and all the unanswered questions regarding optimal care of the disease. I became interested in the process of how to ask a question, design a research study, and work collaboratively to answer the question. With invested mentorship around me, I started to build my career as a scientist. I have always worked with clinical samples (blood, urine, sputum, etc.), so I have maintained my connection with patients and families, which has made the work incredibly rewarding.

— Terri Laguna, MD

Thinking about the WHY will create the fire behind your research program, and it will help narrow the approach you chose to generate questions, which will be answered by your studies. Knowing your research comes from a compelling interest and passion, and that you can articulate those interests and passions to someone else, allows you to make the best case for the value of your research. Research is driven by studies conducted with fidelity and rigor in order to answer critical questions. However, in order for you to be able to conduct those studies, you need funding, colleagues, research team members, and department leaders who identify with and agree on your projects. If you cannot articulate WHY your TOPIC is of critical importance to your colleagues, let alone to yourself, then your research career will come to a screeching halt.

Some people consider developing a research TOPIC (the WHAT) and passion focus (the WHY) to be essential to drafting your own research mission statement. (We will get to that at the end of this chapter). Whatever gives you clarity to identify your seminal research focus and the reason why it is of fundamental interest to you will lend you greater leverage to move your career forward.

HOW

Once you have identified the TOPIC that you are passionate about (the WHAT) and have determined how it is compelling (the WHY), you need to determine the APPROACH to your research that you like the best (the HOW). Many topics can be approached many ways. Each has merits, and the TOPIC and the APPROACH both need to be a passion of yours in order to engage fully.

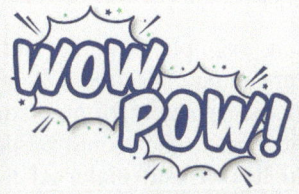

Taylor is a productive assistant professor researcher in the department of family medicine. They made a name for themselves early as a junior faculty for accomplishing and publishing several projects related to the launch of a new Veterans Affairs medical records system. When asking Taylor about the WHAT and WHY of their research passion, they struggled to answer. They explained, "I've always done projects that came from someone knocking at my door to ask me to do them." Now Taylor is faced with the prospect of writing a career development award, and they need to really think through what their WHAT and WHY are. The take-home point is that even if you enter research without a concise mission statement, it is an important step in becoming an independent investigator. Through reflection and developing their own mission statement, Taylor determined what types of projects they wanted to do, as well as knowing when to say "yes" or "no, thanks" to people when asked to take on new work.

What approach do you love to use?

- Biophysics?
- Molecular biology?
- Animal studies?
- Clinical studies?
- Clinical trials?
- Epidemiology?
- Observational?
- Qualitative?
- Implementation sciences?
- Advocacy work?

Let's take an example. You are interested in malaria research. You are passionate about it because of its global health implications, especially for pregnant women. There are many ways that a researcher could be interested in malaria research, global health, and maternal health but approach their research programs in starkly different manners. Someone may be interested in clinical studies that involve fieldwork in endemic regions, partnering with international health ministries. Someone else may be interested in the biology of malarial diseases by studying hepatic cell function. A third person may be interested in the differences in gene expression during the parasitic life cycle stages. All of these fit within the research TOPIC of malaria and within the PASSION of global health and maternal health, but the APPROACH is grounded in a researcher's interest in a style of scientific research. Each of these is valid. The approach you pick is based on your training, your interest, your institution's support for your approach, and your collaborators. However, fundamentally, these approaches must be picked first based on your interest in that mode of science. If you love bench work, you should probably not focus solely on observational research projects. If you want to run a clinical trial, tissue culture work and mosquito microdissection will feel unsatisfying. Additionally, your APPROACH will affect the departments that you would join and the types of funding for which you can apply.

WHO

Finally, after you have determined your topic (the WHAT) and approach (the HOW) that focuses on your passions (the WHY), then you must determine the people (the WHO) you need to answer the questions raised in your research. There will be times when you are unable to do research in a specific manner, or with a specific team, that is ideal. However, when you are reflecting on these questions, you should identify what you really would prefer. It may be hypothetical, but it should be your vision of a scientific utopia. This will help you determine what type of research position you like within academics. Collaborator? Co-investigator? Lead member of large projects across departments and schools? Director of a core laboratory? Leader of a small research lab or team?

To think about the WHO, you need to parse your ideal roles: (Fig. 2.1a–c)

You as an *individual*: How do you yourself want to conduct research? When we initially train in biomedical sciences, most often the topic and the approach are dictated by our mentors. We do a lot of work, the collection and summary of the data, ourselves. However, once we transition to an inde-

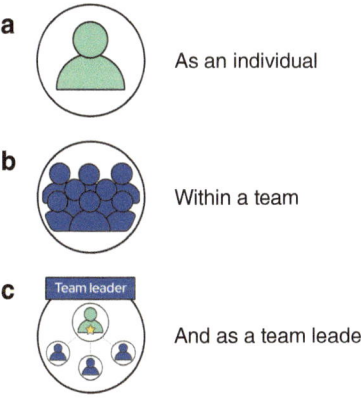

a   As an individual

b   Within a team

c   Team leader   And as a team leader

FIGURE 2.1 (**a**) Individual. (**b**) Team. (**c**) Team lead

pendent investigator, this may be the first time we get to think about how we want to expand or modify that role. Will you lead the development of new research ideas? Execute the studies? Collect the data? Write the results for publication? As a research leader, you need to think about what you enjoy the most and also what is required for your job. Typically, as a principal investigator it is expected that you think about new research ideas and determine how best to execute those projects. However, some researchers will always love "being at the bench" and will want to have time to both think about their current and new projects as well as execute some of the real work that is a part of answering research questions. Other researchers learn that they love writing and speaking and will choose to leverage those talents in their research career. Focus on those talents and wants that you have as an individual and allow the other components of conducting research to be delegated to a colleague or a lab member, or become shared responsibilities.

You as a *team member*: As a team member, you need to consider the way you want to join a group. When you are a team member, with shared responsibilities across a project, you are not the leader. You are completing work that is a component of a larger project. This style of research often occurs in larger, clinically based studies, big data studies, and federal program projects. Each core may have a lead within it, but fundamentally the subprojects all feed into a larger purpose. At times you will be critical to the projects' goals, and at times you will be minimally involved. How can you add to that work over time? Does being a useful participant in a larger project seem satisfying, or do you dislike that because you are not the leader of the project and may not be managing its overall progress? What are the ways that you can fit in best as a participant without necessarily being the director of that work? How will you still be assured that your voice is heard? Reflection on this style of research is important. Your work is critical, but you are joining the project goals rather than charging it forward on your command.

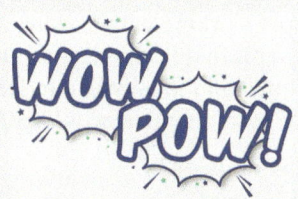

Helena is a post doc working in her mentor's lab. Her mentor is an international expert on plant biology. In thinking about a junior faculty position and a first grant submission, her mentor told her: "I'll sketch out your grant aims and you can write it from there, I know where the field is headed." An all-too common trap for junior women investigators to fall into is to conduct research in line with their mentor for too long and miss opportunities to launch their own ideas as an independent investigator. When thinking about the WHO of your research career, it is important to reflect on whether you want to be an independent investigator, separate from your mentor, or whether you want to be your mentor's co-investigator for the duration of your career. Helena took some time to reflect on her research mission and draw up a proposal that aligned and explained her mission, her previous experiences, and her planned next steps. She then scheduled a meeting with her mentor to discuss her long-term goals towards being an independent investigator; this allowed her mentor to see her as having individual goals and research ideas.

You as a *team leader*: An individual researcher completes all of the work, from the spark of the idea to the publication of the science, only if she has no one else on the team. That style of research is almost unheard of. Science and scientific pursuits are a team sport. There may be things that you enjoy completing on your own, but if you are successful, you will have other people working with and for you that you need to lead as a team. With that in mind, you should determine how many people you would ideally like to lead.

What level of team member would you want?

- High school volunteers?
- Postdoctoral fellows?
- Technicians?
- Research associates?
- Staff scientists?

How will you hire your next team member? What do you like to do less as a researcher, or have less skill in than others? People who have those skills are who you should work with or hire. How will you determine if someone is executing poorly on her projects and not completing her work? How will you support her, or if needed let her go? How will you choose to delegate work? Direct members of your research team in their individual work and project goals? How will you guide their time management and establish project deadlines and target goals?

How many people would you want to oversee? An intimate group of two or three, so that you are hands-on and directly involved? A large group of 25, where subgroups form and are led from within? Again, this is thinking about ideals, your scientific utopia, where you and your team are in their best balance. You should determine a perfect research group for you as a team member, and a team leader, so that your individual strengths are maximized. It will allow you to enjoy working with a group each and every day.

I.CAN'T.EVEN.

OK, so this is a lot to think about. We know. Do not quit on us now. You are a woman scientist, and you can take it. Keep in mind, the answers to the questions above may change over time. That is ok! We have been conditioned to think of our careers as a straight line, or a ladder to climb. The reality is usually (and thankfully) a bit more interesting. Career paths can look like a game of Chutes and Ladders, a sine wave, or moving across a lattice.

Read a little Walt Whitman to remind yourself that you can contradict yourself. And you do contain multitudes. But you need a starting point, and thinking through these questions, writing down your ideas and plans means that you are beginning a mindful and purposeful journey. The next steps in this chapter may help further illuminate the questions you have just considered.

When Things Do Not Go as Planned

Science is often a journey, and our own processes of determining what type of science we want to do can also be a journey. Some scientists start out on one path and then realize they need to shift to a different one. Some scientists need more time to determine which path is right for them. Sometimes one's scientific interests end up much different than one thought they would, or should, be. We hope that the tools and strategies in this chapter will help you engage in reflection to be sure you are on the path that is right for you. Below we include stories from two amazing women scientists to illustrate that diverging from a planned path can be necessary to get to the right path.

I took a long and perfectly circuitous route to finding my love for the study of media influences on health. Although media effects was the topic that peaked my interest in a research career, I dropped it immediately upon admission to graduate school. It just wasn't the kind of thing supported by PhD programs in Psychology at the time, and I saw my future as a tenured Psychology professor at a top ten research university. It was more than a decade before the breadcrumbs that I dropped along my career path led me back "home." My undergraduate thesis tested the influence of exposure to films that pair violence with sexual themes (think Brian DePalma's Dressed to Kill or the scads of horror films featuring a scantily clad babysitter) on young men's attitudes toward sexual violence. I had the fantastic opportunity to work with experts in the area who had a grant on the topic and let me join their lab team. It was a fun,

dynamic group and I made lifelong friends and colleagues. In gradu-
ate school, I turned to a focus on the nuts and bolts of cognition and
behavior, studying how social contexts shape self-perceptions, and
the importance of how people process social information in deter-
mining the outcome of this process. I maintained this focus when I
began my research career, spending 6 years in that tenure-track posi-
tion I had dreamed of. I loved thinking about these deep theoretical
issues, but I lost interest in the methods involved in testing them, and
the published literature in psychology was becoming dry and unin-
teresting to me. But I didn't know how to have a research career
outside of academia. I learned of an opening at RAND Corporation,
a non-profit research institute, when several colleagues pushed me to
apply. Coming to RAND was like being a kid in a candy store, but
one who gets hungrier with every piece she samples. There were lots
of things to which I was able to apply my knowledge, and ample
opportunity test new theories. But the one that really grabbed me was
a project examining the influence of alcohol advertising on underage
drinking. It was like coming home. I realized that much of what I had
been studying for the dozen or so years since I turned away from
media research was highly relevant, and that I had grown as a
researcher in ways that allowed me to bring a unique perspective to
the problem. I was captivated, and by drawing on contacts from that
lab where I worked as an undergrad, I was able to put together a
team and find funding for more work on the topic, this time looking
at how media influences adolescent sexual behavior. I had come
back to where I started, but with a new perspective informed and
enriched by a diverse set of experiences and colleagues I had encoun-
tered along the way.
— Rebecca Collins, PhD

The roadblocks I have encountered in my career have been of both
a personal and professional nature, and I could say the first road-
block I stumbled into was pretty much at the start of my career, as
I was completing graduate school. The world class training I
received put me on an NIH funded academic research career tra-
jectory, however given some personal and professional priorities
the next logical step of a postdoctoral fellowship was neither fis-
cally nor vocationally suitable for me. I remember the department
hallway party immediately after my dissertation defense, when
asked what I would be doing next and my answer of "I'm not sure
yet" was met with dumbfounded silence by those who could not
imagine any next step other than subsequent academic roles and
other mechanisms of grant funding. The environment where I
received my training, and those guiding me through it, were not
adequately equipped to represent the full range (or even beyond a
narrow range) of career possibilities available to someone like me

who was not fulfilling the traditional expectation of a newly minted Ph.D. So my celebration was dampened somewhat by an undercurrent of terrified uncertainty, knowing I was ready to start this great career ahead but not having much of a clue where to start beyond the one single path I was being presented with. I began working around this roadblock by reaffirming my priorities, my professional interests, and my abilities. I was confident in all of those things and believe being straightforward and unapologetic about them helped me move forward. I started looking up and reaching out to people whose work I admired over the course of my education and asked them about their own journeys to that point, and if they were working on something I found appealing how I could have a role. I have continued to use this strategy throughout my career, while not to overcome subsequent roadblocks but to move into positions best suiting my interests and needs at any given time. Some have been more traditional and what my academic mentors would have expected while others have been less so. But all have ultimately lead me to where I am now, so I am thankful for the all challenges and experiences I have encountered over the course of my career.
— *Marsha Lopez, PhD*

What Do You Value? What Are Your Strengths?

When you have clarified what topic area you are engaged in studying and why, the method you love to approach research, and the individual and team-approach you want to execute this work, you also need to step back and think about what it is that you value. Although it may seem to make more sense to think your values and strengths before your research topic and approach, doing them in this order allows you to understand best how to be a researcher. Your values and strengths inform how you will approach your work and how you will rock your science. These values and strengths are innate to you and should not waiver significantly with time. They are the context with which you approach life, and within your life, your work. They will be merged with your research passions to help define your best working style. What you value is something that permeates your life. This is the individual context that you bring to your research topic and approach.

Whether or not this is too touchy-feely for you, this self-reflection will create a sound foundation for your career approach in research. This self-reflection will form an individual academic development plan. That plan will include your: values and strengths, time management style, long-term goals and approach to those goals, and mission statement.

What do you value? What do you hold yourself accountable for or accountable to?

To help determine what you value, you need to reflect on who you are (Fig. 2.2).

- What words would you use to describe yourself?
- What are your qualities?
- What are your strengths?

There are many ways that we describe ourselves. We often create a list of our characteristics or identities to describe ourselves—gender, position within a family, religion, race or ethnicity, where we live, and where we grew up. However, in this self-reflection, pivot from these labels to reflect on your

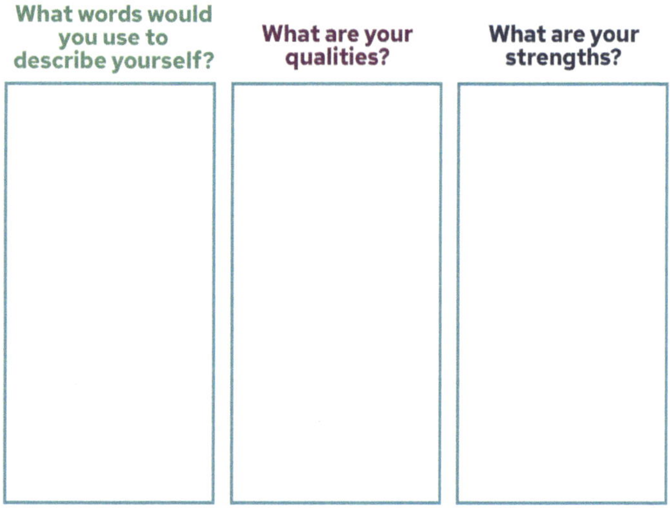

What words would you use to describe yourself?	What are your qualities?	What are your strengths?

FIGURE 2.2 Who are YOU?

own qualities and abilities. Be honest, not lofty or denigrating. Be clear about what you hold true to, and what you bring to your role as a researcher, scientist, professional, and your life across all contexts. Use a single word for each value, quality, and strength you identify about yourself. A true test of these words is that not only do you define yourself with these words, but others should see these values in you too. They should be obvious and accurate. Write these words down. Really. This list will be your word bank that is "all about you."

Once you have created this list, place the words in rank order. What are your greatest values, a value that touches on all aspects of your life? Do you value hard work? Diligence? Diversity? Service to others? Family? Education? Honesty? What are your greatest strengths? Are you organized? Creative? Diligent? Intuitive? Empathetic? Driven? Relatable? These values and strengths should weave through your work, your practice, and your home life, and again they should speak to the core of who you are, having been consistent for years. There should be up to five things at the top of this list that ring true. They rise above all others.

Take those top five words and expand on what those single words really mean to you. Use these single words that best represent you and leverage them as a launching point for deepening your self-reflection. Write down what each value means and defines about you. Try to keep these descriptions succinct—a paragraph is more than enough. Do not just describe why these values accurately reflect you, but also explain why these values are also the most important thing about and for you.

Here is an example of a value. Grit. This description—stick-to-it-ness—is the focus of many books, education tools, and discussions around the dinner table. However, grit as a value may be different for you than for other academicians. What does it mean to you to have grit? For you, that value may mean you can balance many projects, goals, demands on your time. That value may mean persevering in research during a poor funding climate. That value may mean continuing to develop a clinical site despite setbacks in space acquisition, staffing, and the goals of administrators. More broadly, the value of grit may be pushing forward in leadership roles despite being a greater and greater minority in a male-dominated field. By thinking about your own values, and your own strengths, you should be ready to merge your passions in research with your values and strengths next to define your best working style to execute on your lifelong research programs.

Tools to Consider

For some of us, it is challenging to think through strengths and values without a way to assess or evaluate ourselves. There are tools out there that can help with this. We do not specifically endorse any of these, but put them out to consider if you would like some options to assess yourself and get feedback to help shape your understanding of yourself.

1. Meyers-Briggs: The Meyers-Briggs Type Indicator has been around a long time. The assessment tool provides you feedback on dimensions of your personality and traits, including whether you tend to be more introverted or extroverted, more spontaneous, or more of a planner.
2. The Enneagram: The Enneagram has also been around a long time. After taking an assessment you learn where you are centered among nine different "types." A difference in the Enneagram is that your type typically draws from other types in certain situations, such as when you are under stress. Some people like this more dynamic aspect to the Enneagram in understanding their strengths and weaknesses.
3. The iOPT: The input-output-processing-template has a weird name, but it is a helpful tool in understanding how you like to organize and communicate at work. This tool is often used in the business world and can be helpful in considering how you can best organize and communicate in your lab.
4. The StrengthsFinder: This is a tool that provides you feedback after an assessment on your areas of strength. You can then read more about those strengths and consider how to better leverage them in your work.

What Is Your Work Style? Daily Time Management and Long-Term Tasks

How do work? More specifically, how do you like to work? What is your working style? For many, that is something they have never thought about. For decades we are told how to learn and how to complete our work. In training, we rarely have the opportunity to modify how we execute our work. We show up when we are told to do so. We complete our work in the model of our mentors, or supervisors, our institutions. Only when we are "done" training are we offered the opportunity to think about what works best for us. Now is the time to design your work around your best working style. We often think, "When I'm in charge, things will be different." That time is now. Understanding your own working style will allow you to get things done in an even better manner, more efficiently, and with less long-term fatigue and career burnout.

Think about:

- How do you work? More specifically, how do you like to work?
- Do you take a metered approach to deadlines?
- Do you like the intensity of working up to a deadline?
- Do you like group work or independent work? Shared or individual responsibility?
- In what ways do you think about your work? Approach a task?
- Are you a "digital" or "analog" person?
  - Do you see things visually?
  - Do you remember to-do lists only if you write them down?
  - Say them out loud?
  - Use a digital calendar?
- Do you keep your inbox at zero? Like creative chaos?

When you have been honest with how you work, and your preferred working style, then you can approach the best way to manage your time. Time management is not just about how you spend time at work. Time management extends through-out your day and your life. Work is a part of your life. And your life outside of work affects your productivity at work.

Think about:

- What is your best time of day? Are you a night owl? Early bird? Need your first cup of coffee before even getting out of your PJs?
- How do you manage meetings?
- How do you manage menial, boring tasks?
- How do you plan a long-term goal or project?
  - Do you break them down into short-, medium-, and long-term goals with targets?
  - How do you manage your daily work, weekly work, monthly work?
- How do you manage disruption, errors, missed deadlines?
- How do you manage colleagues? Team members? Subordinates?
- How do you manage your office space? Team space? Work away from the office?
- How do you use downtime while commuting? Waiting for a meeting that is starting late? Running late?

Learning your working style, and turning a deliberate focus to time management, you can create a work environment that best supports a strong focus on research. If you think most creatively and critically in the morning hours, leave that time open for scientific reading, planning research projects and proposals, and do not schedule standing meetings that will disrupt that time of day. Two hours in the morning for you may greatly surpass 2 h in the evening for overall productivity.

If disruptions during your day (a phone call, a clinical page, a student who just drops by) really derail you, then close your door or hang a "do not disturb" sign on your entrance. Make an ad hoc meeting less hospitable by not offering a chair to uninvited guests or let them know that they should come back for a scheduled time to discuss a topic that they "just wanted to go over with you." If something is critical, it merits an immediate response, but very often, minor disruptions throughout your day can make your time ineffective. Conversely, if a quiet space with no distractions is too isolating for you, keep your door open. Let yourself go visit your staff or lab members. Let the stimulation of people, sounds, and movement scratch your social itch so that you can return to your focused and creative work renewed.

That are many tasks that we must do as academic researchers that are necessary evils. Paperwork. Progress reports. Updating CVs. Budget management. Travel receipts and reimbursements after a work trip. None of these are items many people relish. However, they must be done. How do you approach work that you would rather put off…indefinitely? Can you break it into smaller chunks, reviewing your budgets monthly so it takes only a little time to keep up? Can you concentrate this work so you have dedicated time to do the repetitive tasks while rewarding yourself with a trip to the coffee shop at the end? Again, think about this, and your ideal, within the context of your day, your week, month, and year, and within the context of research projects being done by you and your research team.

Define your preferred time management style and also your research and academic career goals. Highlight where you want to be in 5–10 years and the steps you will need to take to get there. Think about your long-term work, and break it down into more manageable pieces remembering both your daily work style and the ebb and flow of the academic year. Again, write this all down. Do not worry; we know things change, but with at least annual reviews of your individual academic plan, you can see if you are on-track, ahead of the game, or changing course. Honesty in your approach and goals is key to academic and scientific success.

In the context of time management, advice we would give about planning and executing long-term projects is first to learn how long something may actually take. How long is the IRB process at your institution? How challenging is it to set up a new protocol in your laboratory? How do you process interview transcripts to be able to code them for themes?

Next, we would advise that you think about projects in reverse chronologic order. A catchy phrase for this is "begin with the end in mind." When does your project need to end? At the end of a project, what are the products that you will have created? A new teaching module? Several peer-reviewed research papers? The pilot data for a new grant application? Then, with that end in mind, work backward. Take that long-term project and break it into smaller, medium-sized pieces. What will you do the first 6 months, the second 6 months? Then finally, within those smaller pieces, what will you do this month, this week, and today?

Smaller pieces are do-able. Large projects can be so overwhelming that you stagnate. Rather than saying today you will write a grant, perhaps today is the day you review currently funded grants in your area of interest. Next, you do literature reviews of key investigators in your field. Then, you work on ideas and discuss them with peers and colleagues. The final goal is the same, a grant proposal, but each small piece is manageable and can be balanced with all of the other work required for your academic career and position.

Do Not Forget Self-Care

Keeping good care of your health, mental and physical, is key to effective time management. Someone might say, how do you exercise when there is so much to do? How can you schedule a visit to the doctor for your family members, let alone yourself, when you need to run a meeting, travel for work, or complete revisions for a manuscript? Just like all of the other parts of your work and life, your health needs attention too. Without a strong mental focus, and good physical health, it is nearly impossible to attend to the critical thinking needed to do unique and cutting-edge research in academic medicine. However, to ensure that good practices for mental and physical health fit in for your life, you must address these consistently just like another task that is assigned to you through work. You need to rock yourself to rock your science.

Figure out what you need for self-care. A few critical elements are sleep, food, and physical activity. Think carefully and deeply about how you will incorporate healthy habits into your busy life. You want to be in this for the long game, and ignoring these areas is contrary to your goals.

Another important thing to consider are your self-care/rejuvenation strategies if you hit the wall in the middle of the day and cannot concentrate. Will you take a walk around the block? Do a 20-min yoga session? Grab a cup of coffee? Read some poetry? Begin to build a toolbox you can turn to when you run out of steam and need to recharge and get back to work.

Further, consider ways you will treat yourself when you achieve accomplishments. It is important to note you should recognize your own accomplishments that represent what you have *done*, such as submitting a paper, grant, or presentation proposal. Do not reserve your treats for just things that get accepted or awarded. You did your first talk at a national meeting? You survived your first grant rejection? You just submitted a manuscript you have been working on, on time and on your own deadline? Time for a……massage? Lunch date with a friend? Shopping trip to your favorite place? Leaving work early to take an extra-long bike ride? You fill in the blanks...

A Note About Haters

There will always be haters in science, and in every other field. They are not worth your time. The less time we and you can spend on them, the more time we can spend on our science.

Your Mission Statement

As you come to understand WHAT kind of work you want to do and HOW, you should also draft a mission statement. A mission statement should be a part of your individual academic plan, as it is a common tool used in academic clinical research. This is a statement meant to tie together your goals and your approaches into a cohesive mission. It should be succinct, almost pithy, and fully represent you. Admittedly, it is not easy to write for the first time. But once it is written, it can serve several important purposes.

1. Your mission statement can serve as the foundation of your *"elevator speech."* This "speech" is the 2-minute synopsis of your work. It is called an "elevator speech" because at a moment's notice you should be able to sum up your work quickly, such as if you are riding an elevator with a senior colleague (or a potential philanthropic donor!). You need to finish your speech before the elevator doors open. We discuss the use of the elevator speech at national conferences in Chap. 5. Another time you will need your "elevator speech" is at Thanksgiving—your second cousin never really wants to know the details of your work—just the gist.

2. Your mission statement becomes a *guidepost* for figuring out when to say "yes" and when to say "no." When you are asked to do something in your department, if the requested task is consistent with your mission statement, you know a "yes" is within reach. If not, then you have a solid rationale for declining that task.

3. Your mission statement becomes your *image* or your *identity*, and looking at it should feel like looking in the mirror. Just as your individual academic development plan should be reviewed at least annually, your mission statement should be reviewed periodically as well. Your mission statement will be a statement you return to, yearly, or quarterly, or even weekly at some points in your career, to be sure that it still represents your mission. To help with that self-evaluation, your mission statement should be saved as a word document with a date, so that as you update it you can "save as" with a new date.

Here is an example mission statement: *I hope to improve the quality of chronic illness care for adolescents, especially vulnerable teens, by improving adherence to evidence-based guidelines in primary care settings for ADHD.* Short. Sweet. To the point. A distillation of her WHAT and WHY. This mission statement provides information on:

- The study population: Adolescents, especially vulnerable teens with ADHD
- The approach: quality of care
- The specific area of focus: evidence-based guidelines

Thus, for this faculty member, if asked to be on a committee to review clinic adherence to primary care guidelines on chronic illnesses, she would know that this falls well within her mission. If she were asked to help write a paper on adult surgical guidelines, that would be a good one to decline.

For some people, a mission statement is just too hard to put into words at first. Maybe your doctoral work differed from your postdoctoral focus, or you did research as a medical student that is different than what you are doing now. Not all of our research careers are linear, so a visual image or model can sometimes represent and provide more explanation of where your central mission may lie than simple text. In addition to representing your areas of interest, you can fill in key methods that you like to use or topic areas that you love. This is both a merger of your mission (WHAT and WHY) with your approach (HOW). Figure 2.3 represents an image describing a research path from PhD to post doc to junior faculty, including relevant publications and areas of interest. This was created by Jennifer Whitehill, PhD (thanks Jen!). This image helped shape a mission statement for this scientist's future and her academic development plan. Even if you have an image representing your interests, it is still important to have a key centralized area of focus you can describe to yourself and others.

Areas of Interest & Main Fellowship Projects

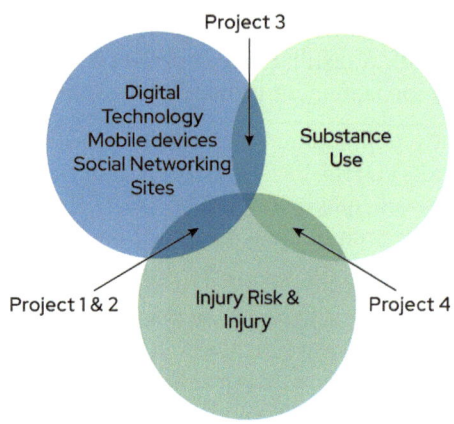

Current Goals

1. Build experience in research on new media technology and injury prevention
2. Expand research from intentional injury to unintentional injury

Future Goal

1. Policy Relevant research that addresses issues that span all 3 bubbles above

FIGURE 2.3 Dr. Jennifer Whitehill's visual mission statement

Take-Home Points

Well-executed research requires a lot from us. Therefore, it is critical to understand what drives you to conduct research.

Before you know your science, you need to know yourself.

To keep doing your science, you need to take care of yourself.

You need to identify *what* you are passionate about in research, *how* you want to execute that research, *why* you love it so, and *who* you want to bring into your team to push your research to its best. It is equally important to understand what your own values and strengths are.

These values and strengths define who you are, and within that context, determine your best approach to research and a career in academic medicine.

Bringing your values and strengths to your everyday will clarify your working style and a time management system that is ideal for who you are.

Homework
- Develop your individual academic development plan:
  - Determine what your own values are.
  - Rank these and pick the top five to further define and describe about you.
  - Identify your strengths.
  - Project where you want to be in 10 years.
  - Develop intermediate goals (1, 3, and 5 year goals).
  - Use your introspection on your own time management to plan your intermediate goals.
  - Identify what skills and support you will need to achieve these goals.
  - Identify who will help guide you to achieve these goals.
  - Write a mission statement representing your goals and approaches, using images if needed to shape the text-based statement.

Chapter 3
Your Team: Mentors, Staff, Colleagues, and Mentees

In this chapter we will focus on your team, representing the most immediate connected circle of your socioecological model (SEM). Chapter 1 defined the socioecological model, and Chap. 2 considered your role as an individual scientist within that model. In this chapter, we will consider your innermost circle, or your WomenRockScience team. We will consider your team to be the people who work in your immediate or virtual vicinity, either in your research group or directly supporting your research group in real-time or online. Your team includes your mentoring/oversight team (people who oversee your work), your research team (people who you oversee), collaborators (people working alongside you, such as peers), and colleagues (your close network). Within the SEM, these folks have a direct effect on your research career and how much you can rock your science.

Your Mentors

We will start with your mentors, who are critical to your success as a scientist. You will again note that when we use a third person pronoun, we will use a female pronoun. However,

M. A. Moreno, R. Katzenellenbogen, *Women Rock Science*, https://doi.org/10.1007/978-3-031-48418-6_3

we want to recognize that people across all genders can be excellent mentors. A first myth that we would like officially to "bust" is that you only need one mentor. To be successful and happy, you will need a few mentors who can serve different roles. Some of these relationships may be more formal, others may evolve into mentoring without either party making it official. Some people will fulfill more than one type of mentoring for you, and others' involvement will be more focused or limited.

Mentoring is different from other relationships, such as advising, coaching, advocating, or being a role model. We will unpack this a bit to demonstrate their differences. **Advising** is typically a time-focused, directive relationship within a specific domain of your professional development. For example, college advisors helped you figure out what classes to take. **Coaching** helps you hone a skill through training, practice, and review. For example, basketball coaches run drills and scrimmages at practices and orchestrate team plays during a game, giving feedback in real time to their players. **Advocating** is providing you support, typically supporting you openly to those above you on the organizational chart at your institution. For example, your division head may be an advocate who helps communicate your needs to your department chair. Being a **role model** is embodied in people whom you look up to; their work is what you model your career on, and therefore that relationship entails more passive observation.

An ideal mentor encompasses many or all of these qualities, but a mentor's role also goes beyond those listed above. A mentoring relationship is more complex, implies a deeper investment on the part of the mentor, and is usually a longer relationship. They guide rather than direct or merely support. Thus, their relationship should be truly altruistic and should function to aid you in finding your own "best" so you can then do your best.

Meaningful Moments

I tend to subdivide academic career development into three phases—training, climbing, and building. Training is the part during which you open yourself to the process while others have the responsibility for guiding your development and ensuring you reach basic professional milestones. While training is hard and the expectations are high for those balancing the triad of academic responsibilities (clinical, teaching, and research) there is a nurturing structure that moves you towards autonomy and the light is almost always visible at the end of the tunnel.

—Maria Trent, MD, MPH

A few types of mentors include:

1. *Primary research mentor*: This person has the greatest input into your research career and the greatest stake in your success. This person's work likely has some overlap with yours, so a key part of the relationship over time will be your mentor providing you teaching and guidance while allowing you to evolve as an independent scientist.

   Most people meet with their primary research mentor weekly or every other week during the early career phase. Often this frequency will decrease over a period of years, and usually with ongoing discussion at designated check ins.

   Many people find that over time, the relationship someone has with their primary research mentor may evolve into one more like a close colleague. However, that lingering goal of a primary research mentor making decisions based on what is best for you (and not for them) should still flavor the relationship.

2. *Research project mentor*: If you are doing a project that requires a specific skillset that your mentor does not have, for example, a specific test to be done as part of the project or a complicated statistical analysis, you may have a research project mentor. This person may play a more limited role in your career as they are mainly focused on one of your projects. However, these are scientists whose role sometimes evolves over time if you work well with them.

   You may find that you meet with your project mentor weekly during the project. Afterward the project is complete, consider scheduling a follow-up meeting to discuss how the project went and get feedback. If you find that your style matches well with that person, consider meeting with her intermittently to keep this person in your larger circle of mentors.

3. *Clinical mentor:* Clinical scientists often find it helpful to have a clinician mentor. This person can be helpful both with providing clinical role modeling and teaching, and keeping you interested and invested in clinical medicine. This mentor may also help by discussing research ideas to be sure your projects are in the realm of clinical relevance.

4. *Career mentor*: A career mentor is someone who can keep an eye on the big picture of where your career is and where it is headed. This person can truly embody the SEM perspective and can help you to consider your involvement in different arenas of your career SEM. For example, this mentor may talk with you about whether you should be taking on fewer local committee responsibilities so you have time for larger scale work with your national scientific organization. You may find it helpful to ask your career mentor to review your mission statement and your SEM model.

5. *Near-peer mentor*: While many of us think of mentors as being among the "gray hairs," there is much to be said for having near-peer mentors. A near-peer mentor is typically a step or two ahead of where you are in your career. So, for a PhD student, a near-peer mentor may be a senior student or post doc. For a medical resident or fellow, a near-peer

mentor may be a junior faculty member. These mentors can often provide you with helpful advice and counsel on preparing for what is next, as they are currently in that next place. Their advice can often be quite practical, examples of things we have learned from near-peer mentors were how to save money on conference travel, or how to navigate working with a grumpy administrator.

6. *Cheerleader mentor*: Most of us know someone we have worked with that is incredibly positive. This person can usually turn lemons into lemonade, and so you walk away from an interaction with this person Just.Feeling.Better. This person's area of work may have little overlap with yours, but it is her attitude and approach that is her strength. Seek out your cheerleader mentor after a paper rejection, an unfunded grant, or a challenging let down. This person will keep you going.

It is worth noting that sometimes a mentor may start in one role, such as a project mentor, and evolve to fill another role, such as primary mentor. It is also possible that a single mentor may fill more than one mentoring role for you. Finally, you may worry that no one will want to be a mentor, or specifically your mentor, because you may worry that nothing is gained by them from such an altruistic act. Have no fear. Many people enjoy and benefit from mentoring, and we discuss some of the benefits of being a mentor in Chap. 7.

Finding Your Mentors

Meaningful Moments
The greatest privilege of being a leader in academic medicine is working with trainees and early stage investigators on their path to independence. They have incredible ideas, and helping them put pieces together for their projects and teams is rewarding. I get so much out of mentoring—it is very much a two-way process.
—Ruanne Barnabas MBChB, DPhil

To find the members of your mentoring circle, we as scientists can rely on...what else but science! First, consider studies that show seeking and finding your own mentors is associated with a more productive relationship compared to having a mentor assigned to you. Seeking out your own mentors does take some work, but evidence shows it is worth it. (And who are we to go against the evidence, right?) The process of finding mentors should lead to a goal product of having mentors. We would also argue that the process in and of itself leads to benefits.

In order to find your mentors, you can use similar approaches as one would with a research project. The steps include the following:

1. **Develop an initial proposal**: In this stage you will consider what types of mentors you want and need. You can use your mission statement from Chap. 2's homework, or your draft SEM from Chap. 1's homework, to identify areas of your work in which you would benefit from specific mentorship. Some specific questions to ask yourself include:
   (a) What areas of science do you want mentors to come from or represent?
   (b) Are there specific project questions or requests you have at this time?
   (c) Are there particular career path questions on the horizon for which you would benefit from a mentor's support?

   Develop this initial list or document, and save it so that you can return to it at different points in your training or career. Your mentoring needs may change over time, but you can return to your own framework each time you want to consider adding a mentor to your circle. Each time you update the document, save it with the new date so you know which version is most current. If you are saving this document in a cloud-based format, you may want to save each version of your list with dates, so that you do not lose your initial ideas and the opportunity to see how your questions and needs have evolved over time.

This part of the process benefits you by using your mission statement and SEM from Chap. 2. You may find that as you navigate this process, your mission or areas of passion or SEM evolve. Thus, keep in mind that you should update those documents as you navigate this process. This step also ensures that you are taking stock of your areas of interest and aligning possible mentors with your actual needs.

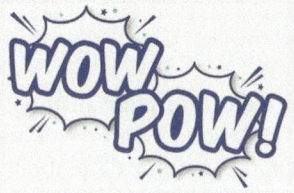

Eliana graduated with a PhD in clinical psychology, and she is now a post doc at a different university. Her PhD mentor, Jane, is a psychiatrist who has focused her career on depression medication interventions. Eliana's dissertation focused on ways to improve adherence to a particular depression medication. For her postdoctoral fellowship, Eliana is currently planning a project to pilot test a complementary medicine intervention for depression. She has identified a family practice physician with complementary medicine expertise as a project mentor. Eliana was concerned to tell Jane about her new project, fearing that her mentor would not approve of her new focus on complementary treatments. She created a proposal document describing how she planned to integrate her previous expertise and new research directions, and she shared it with Jane. To Eliana's relief, Jane was supportive and appreciative of being kept in the loop. Eliana continues to stay in touch with Jane who has been helpful in thinking about her career, and in navigating some tough clinical scenarios. She considers Jane to now be both a career mentor and a clinical mentor. Eliana also spends time with a junior faculty member in the lab, Keshan, who is enthusiastic and supportive of having Eliana there. Keshan has provided valuable advice about how to make the most of a post doc and how to plan ahead for success as a junior faculty. Thus, Eliana views Keshan as both a cheerleader mentor and a near-peer mentor.

2. **Create a data collection plan**: In this stage you will consider how to track your mentor-seeking process and findings. You will want to enter data about potential mentors and what happened when you contacted them. Some people use a spreadsheet-based data collection approach, others use a more narrative format on a document. Either way, you will want to decide what information is important to you to track. For example, you may want to keep track of the areas of interest for that faculty member, or her department/division. Some people keep track of dates they reached out to each person, and when the person replied. This can be helpful to track your progress over time and to have a sense of how rapidly the faculty member responds to emails. Note: Excessive delays in email response can be a marker for being overworked, overwhelmed, or poorly organized, which may help you to know what to expect in responsiveness if you worked with her. You may also want to include an area where you can add people who are referred to you by others. Decide how you want to label these variables and again save it with the date. This will be a "living" document that you will be returning to and updating. An example spreadsheet is below.

Name	Topic area	Contact info	How found	Date emailed	Date responded	Meeting	Notes
Jane Smith	Epidemiology	smith@ xx.edu	University website	1-Mar	1-May	1-Jul	Too hard to get a hold of, may be good career mentor?
Julia Brighton	Health Services	brighton@ xx.edu	Referred by Prof Smith	5-Jul	6-Jul	13-Jul	Good overlap in my topic area, very responsive
Faye Kamp	Health Services	kamp@ xx.edu	Referred by Erik	5-Jul	13-Jul	19-Jul	Specific expertise in maternal health, may be helpful on current project

This part of the process benefits you in creating this document of people, or an environmental scan of those around you. You may find you return to this documentation in the future. This could be months, or even years, later. This document often reflects who is around and available to you as possible colleagues or collaborators, and so your tracking and notes may pay off in ways you can't anticipate.

3. **Create a "subject recruitment" plan**: Now that you have a way to enter and manage your data, in this stage you will develop an initial list of potential mentors. This may be from your department website after looking at potential mentors and their areas of interest expressed there. You may also develop a list of potential mentors with topic expertise based on your university website or other sources.

   (a) Keep in mind that some topics have overlap across fields, so you do not want to miss some important places to look. For example, if you are interested in physical activity interventions for pediatric obesity patients, you may want to look into both pediatric and family medicine approaches, as well as potentially looking within pediatric endocrinology, sports medicine, or physiology, and do not forget about cell biology and biophysics faculty.

   (b) Keep in mind that some mentors may be outside your specific institution. For example, your local department of health may have mentors available. It is also worth considering whether you have local institutions or foundations doing science in your area, such as the Bill and Melinda Gates Foundation or the Institute for Disease Modeling.

   (c) While you are looking for areas of alignment with your research interests, keep in mind the strength that comes from diversity. Considering different perspectives, backgrounds, and expertise while building your team of mentors may greatly contribute to your own success.

4. **Draft your communication**: The next step is to develop your communication plan for reaching out to potential faculty mentors. Typically, this involves an initial email. The email can be used to gauge initial interest and availability to meet. These meetings early-on are a way to get to know potential mentors. They are sometimes called "informational interviews" or colloquially "meet-n-greets."

   (a) For many people, it is more comfortable to set up a meeting to discuss *shared areas of interest* rather than directly asking about the potential of mentorship as the first step. This has advantages in that it puts less pressure on the initial meeting. While a reference to dating is admittedly a bit cheesy, we cannot resist the metaphor that on a first date you typically go for coffee or a meal, and not a weeklong trip. Further, if you meet with the person and find that your work styles are unlikely to be a match, it saves you from trying to figure out how to disengage. An example email is below (Fig. 3.1).

   (b) Draft your email carefully to present yourself as the competent professional science rock star that you are. Use professional titles (professor or Dr.) and a formal introduction. Avoid the words "hi" and "hey," and we do not recommend emoticons or memes at this stage of the game.;)

   (c) Be sure your CV is updated, so that you can send it ahead of time if the faculty member requests it before the meeting, or during, or after the meeting. You may also consider sending your CV at the time you request

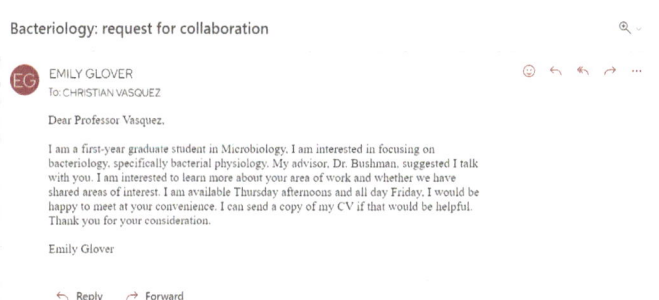

Figure 3.1 Example email to request an informational interview

the meeting, so that the faculty can review it before deciding to meet with you.

(d) If you have already published in the field, some faculty will ask to see a recent abstract or paper, so think ahead about what you would send if you are asked for a recent publication.

5. **Plan your meeting**: These types of introductory meetings typically last about 30–45 min. In that time frame, you will be able to touch on several key points. It is helpful to plan ahead so you know what information you want to share, and so that your questions of this potential mentor can be focused and on point.

(a) Meeting structure

- *Introductions*: Remind the faculty member how and why you identified them and contacted them and remind them who you are (your career stage and your research interests). It is a great idea to use your Elevator Speech that you developed in Chap. 2 to summarize your interests and mission.

- *Ask them to talk about their work*, some potential phrases to consider include (Fig. 3.2):
  - "I'm interested in hearing about your work."
  - "Can you tell me a little about your training and how it led to your area of research focus?"
  - "I'd love to learn about your research."
  - Sometimes the faculty member wants you to talk about your interests first. Be careful not to get carried away and take all the time for your meeting. You already know what you are interested in, so be sure to take some time to find out what this potential mentor is interested in, then you can assess the fit of this person as a mentor. It may be worth practicing what you are going to say ahead of time, you probably want to talk for no more than 5 min. Consider taking your 2-min elevator speech you developed in Chap. 2 and adding a bit more detail.

1. "I'm interested in hearing about your work"

2. "Can you tell me a little about your training and how it led to your area of research focus?"

3. "I'd love to learn about your research."

FIGURE 3.2 Example questions to use during an informational interview

- *Your interests*: Then, the faculty member will typically ask you to talk about your work.

 – If the faculty member does not ask you to talk about your work, that is a pretty big **red flag** suggesting she either is not interested, is not socially adept, or expecting you to fall in line with her work.

  – So long as we are on the topic of **red flags**, another huge red flag is when the faculty member is dismissive of your work and suggests you use the "more advanced methods" that she is using, or even to drop your area of interest and join her lab to work on a current project she is doing. This is usually a sign that she is not a good fit to mentor you (or anyone). Often, these interactions suggest she is looking for someone to work in her lab or work *for* her, and not as a mentee.

- *Areas of shared interest*: At this point, the conversation often turns back to you to describe your areas of interest in a more focused way. Based on the faculty's description of her work, you may call out areas in which your interests overlap with hers.
- *Have 2–3 questions ready*: These may be questions about the faculty member's work, training, or other information that you have garnered from her website or the conversation. It is good to have a few questions ready ahead of time, but you may find that other better questions arise during your conversation so that you do not need the pre-prepared ones.
- *Stay within the time frame of the meeting*: For an initial meeting, you will want to stay within the time allotted to the meeting, which is often 30 min. Even if the faculty you are meeting with does not watch the clock, you should. If you get to the end time, you can mention something like, "I see we are at our end time for this meeting. I'd like to be respectful of both our time and wrap things up." This shows that you are responsible with time and respectful of time limits on meetings. If you wrap up the meeting and feel like there was so much more that could have been said, that is often a good sign that this person may be a good mentor for you.
- *Thanks and wrap up*: Be sure to thank the faculty member for her time to meet with you. At this point, you can consider if you want to ask about her availability to meet again. If there is a specific ask you have in mind you can also feel out that possibility.

- "I've really learned a lot from this meeting that relates to the project I'll be starting soon; do you have availability when I could meet with you again in a few weeks when my project gets started?"
- "I really appreciate this meeting. Would you be able to meet again in the next 2 months so I can run my ideas by you at that point?"

(b) **Send thank you email**: Within a week of your meeting, send a brief thank you email. If you were asked to provide follow-up information, be sure to include that.

Mentor analysis: Many junior scientists will pursue anywhere between 5 and 25 informational interviews or "meet-n-greets." Some of these meetings will lead to productive mentoring relationships. Other meetings will lead to developing collegial relationships and future collaborations. Some meetings will not go anywhere and just be a pleasant (or less pleasant) time spent getting to know another scientist.

If you feel a positive connection to a faculty member during a meeting, you had similar interests, or compatible communication styles, or felt inspired by the ideas discussed in the meeting, set up another meeting in the near future to explore further ideas and plans. If you don't get this sense of connection, do not despair.

If you meet someone, have a positive connection, and are seriously considering working closely with her, but still have some questions, you could do a little more background research. This background research might include asking others who work with her about their experiences or looking into their lab websites. If you were hiring someone to join your group, you would call references. The same can be said here as well. Make sure you are not acting like a private eye or appearing to gossip about a potential mentor, but do consider others' opinions in addition to your own gut feeling.

What Are You Seeking in a Mentor?

Mentors are people, and like all of us they have particular work styles, personalities, and foibles. In choosing to work with a mentor, you will be exposed to all of those elements. You do not have to like or emulate your mentor in total. In fact, seeking mentors who approach things differently than you can be a way to expand your own skillset. And remember, she does not need to be your role model. It is a rare mentor that can fill the shoes of mentor AND role model. Ideally you can derive some learning from who she is as well as how she guides you.

That being said, there are certain characteristics of mentors that are important to consider. These characteristics often include integrity, honesty, trustworthiness, morality, altruism, and a commitment to mentoring. You may want to create your own list of must-haves in these characteristics. Can you accurately evaluate all these on your first meeting? Definitely not. But these characteristics are important to keep in your mind as you get to know a potential mentor.

Lessons from the Lab

When I (Megan) was a junior faculty at a new university, I knew that I would need to do some work to build a mentoring team. In my job contract, I negotiated for a half day off of clinic each week for the first 6 months of my appointment. I used that half day to have 1–2 meetings each week with faculty around my department, the medical school, and the larger campus faculty. I met with dozens of people and made a huge chart of all of my meetings and experiences. Even now, I still have those charts. And occasionally, when I have a new project that would benefit from specific expertise, I can still open up the chart and find the person I remember from over a decade ago. Then I know who to call, and I can reconnect quickly with that person and where our careers have gone, using that as a starting ground for new collaborations on a project.

Further, you want a mentor who will let you develop as an independent scientist. That is important enough to repeat using slightly different terms: you want a mentor who functions as a *guide* rather than a *director.*

You Have Found Some Mentors, Now What?

Time to bust another myth. Once you find a primary mentor, you can relax and let that person take the lead. This is just false and, frankly, foolish. You cannot drive your science from the passenger seat. In any relationship with a mentor, you need to assume that you are in charge of steering the relationship. This is called "mentoring up." You are the one who prompts the next meeting, you make the meeting agenda, and you plan the follow-up. Your mentor is there to guide you, but not to direct your time or micromanage what you do. This is all about your career, not hers. Your active participation is critical and fundamental to the success of mentoring and your science.

In meeting with your mentors, here are some tips for a successful relationship and productive time together (Fig. 3.3):

Risks of Mentorship

Mentorship presents risks. By definition your mentor is taking time to gamble on you and your career, and you are taking a gamble on your mentor's investment in you. Here are a few problems to watch for, and how to prevent or address them.

Problem: Mentors can become disinterested, take on new jobs and roles and no longer have time.

Prevention: Prior to taking on a new mentor and at scheduled intervals (for example, you could schedule yearly or every 6 month reviews of how the mentoring relationship is going), ask your mentor if they anticipate any big career changes on their horizon that would affect your mentoring relationship. This would allow you to plan ahead if changes are coming.

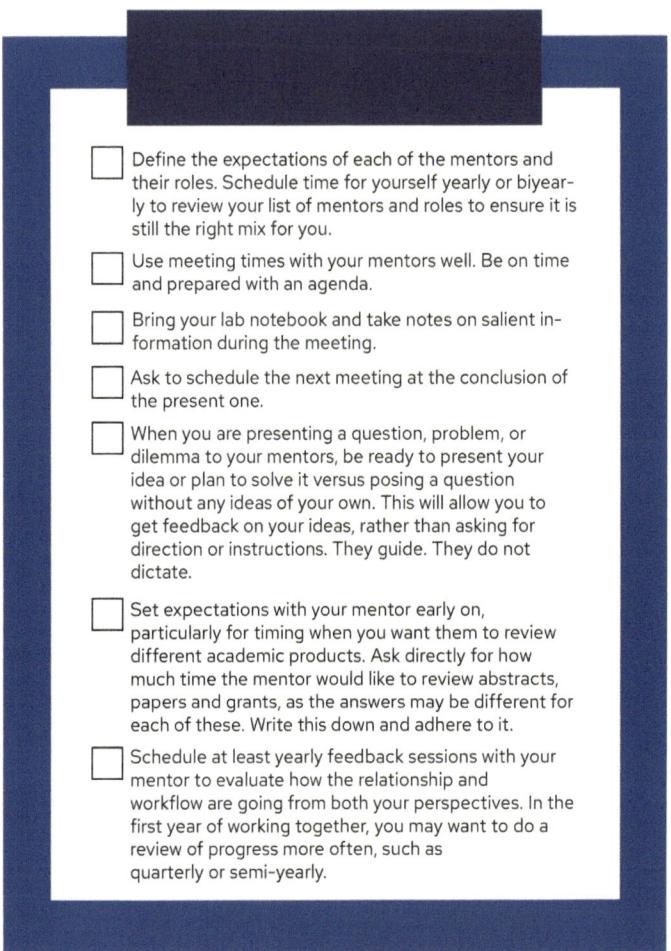

☐ Define the expectations of each of the mentors and their roles. Schedule time for yourself yearly or biyearly to review your list of mentors and roles to ensure it is still the right mix for you.

☐ Use meeting times with your mentors well. Be on time and prepared with an agenda.

☐ Bring your lab notebook and take notes on salient information during the meeting.

☐ Ask to schedule the next meeting at the conclusion of the present one.

☐ When you are presenting a question, problem, or dilemma to your mentors, be ready to present your idea or plan to solve it versus posing a question without any ideas of your own. This will allow you to get feedback on your ideas, rather than asking for direction or instructions. They guide. They do not dictate.

☐ Set expectations with your mentor early on, particularly for timing when you want them to review different academic products. Ask directly for how much time the mentor would like to review abstracts, papers and grants, as the answers may be different for each of these. Write this down and adhere to it.

☐ Schedule at least yearly feedback sessions with your mentor to evaluate how the relationship and workflow are going from both your perspectives. In the first year of working together, you may want to do a review of progress more often, such as quarterly or semi-yearly.

FIGURE 3.3 Checklist for working with your mentor

Intervention: Ask to have a check-in meeting with your mentor focused on your mentoring relationship. During that meeting, express your concerns and ask if you can collaborate on a solution. One solution may be adding another co-mentor who has more time to offer.

Problem: Mentors can foster over-dependency and overlook your career goals. Thus, mentees can become "clones" of their mentors rather than independent investigators. These scenarios may include if your work closely aligns with your mentors, and it is hard to distinguish whose work belongs to whom. Another scenario is if you are working with a mentor who is not interested in your ideas, but is interested in telling you her ideas. Another possible scenario is if you are working with a mentor who keeps telling you to work on her studies and not your own.

Prevention: Schedule check-ins (quarterly or twice a year) as part of ongoing meetings with your mentor that focus on the big picture of your path to independence. Ask your mentor for feedback and guidance on how to continually take steps to develop yourself as an independent investigator.

Intervention: When a situation has evolved such that a mentee has become overly reliant upon or dependent upon a mentor, the fault usually lies in both parties. The mentor has failed to foster independence, and the mentee has failed to move herself forward with her own ideas and taking ownership of them. This situation can be improved or resolved with transparent and frank conversations, but often these situations require the input of others. Some mentors do not see it as a problem if a mentee is basically just doing her work for the mentor's benefit. Involvement of the career mentor, or a leader in one's own division or department can help moderate the situation. This is also when a group meeting is very helpful. A third-party perspective, potentially from your career mentor or your division head as an advocate, can help intervene on your behalf as a mentee. In some cases, involvement of human resources or a campus representative may be needed to ensure that appropriate processes are in place and followed.

Problem: A mentor can take credit or ideas from mentees.

Prevention: This is a lowly behavior, and very hard to address as a mentee. Thus, prevention is critical. Focus on identifying people who have done this before and screening them out. Talking to past mentees before fully committing to a mentor is one way to get a sense of this.

Intervention: This is another situation that benefits from seeking counsel or help. Talking with your career mentor, your near-peer mentors, or your division/department leadership can help you identify the best path to address this. It does not hurt to have excellent record keeping of your science to document your ideas and progress if called upon to do so.

Problem: A mentor demonstrates behavior that is inappropriate or unprofessional.

Prevention: There may be no way to prevent this from happening; however, in no way should you assume fault or blame on yourself if it does.

Intervention: Do not be silent. Document the behavior as soon as possible after it takes place. Find people you trust to talk with and figure out what steps need to be taken as soon as possible. Above all, do not be silent. This merits being said twice. Your campus or institution will have people you can contact about this, and processes to follow. These may include human resources, campus safety, campus police, or a university ombudsperson. Know them all to find the support you need.

Meaningful Moments

The biggest mistake I made in my career was believing that I would not be treated differently than my white, non-Hispanic male colleagues. As I progressed through fellowship and my junior faculty years, I naively assumed that racism, sexism, and discrimination would not impact me. Unfortunately, I found out very quickly that was not the case. As a Latinx, gay, women in academic medicine, I have had to advocate for myself and find my voice very quickly, as I have had to overcome the impacts of harassment and discrimination. I learned the importance of calling out inappropriate behavior and continuing to pursue accountability for it even when it may be dismissed by leadership. This was not easy to learn and even harder to put into practice; however, I can't stress enough the importance of accountability for bad behavior and also serving as a role model to others who are subject to the same sort of discrimination. It is never appropriate, and it is never OK to let it go.

— Terri Laguna, MD

Your Research Lab and Team

Your research team includes your research staff, co-investigators, and mentees who help you get your work done on a day-to-day basis. There are several different structures of research labs and teams. A few common ones include:

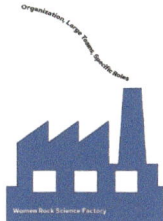

Large labs and teams: Being part of a large research team can be analogous to being part of an efficient machine or factory. These large teams may be within organizations or centers within an academic center. Large teams often have team members with specific roles, such as data collection, or IRB management. These teams may work with one PI, or more than one PI whose work has similarities in methods or topic.

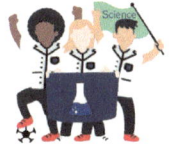

Medium-size labs and teams: Being part of a medium-size research team can be like being part of a sports team. These teams require organization and an understanding of the team culture in order to be productive.

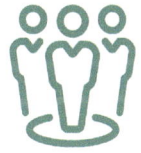

Small labs and teams: Being part of a small research team can be like being part of an elite squad. There is often more day-to-day communication, but the need for structure is no less than any other size.

Regardless of the size of the research lab or team, an organizational structure is needed. These structures determine how the work flows within the team, and what type of communication is expected when decisions need to be made or problems come up in a project. These structures also help shape the culture of that team or lab, as the structure often represents the value or vision of the PI. Three common types of structures may include:

1. *The pyramid*: Similar to businesses and companies, the pyramid structure gives a clear sense of how decisions and power flow. In the pyramid structure, the PI is at the top, senior staff or managers are just below the PI, and these folks manage the work of staff who engage in the daily tasks of research.

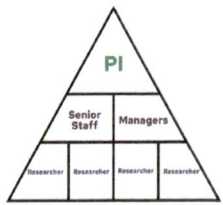

2. *The UN*: Some research labs are built with shared leadership models similar to the United Nations (UN). In this structure, one team member may be a lead on one project but be a staff member for another.

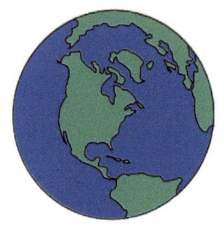

3. *The specialized team*: Some research labs are built with individuals who each have an area of work and specialization and contribute that type of work on each project. In this model, the workflow is driven by what type of work is needed and which individual has expertise to do it.

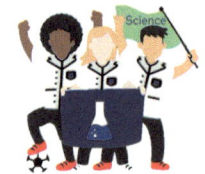

Setting Expectations for Your Team

When setting the expectations for work from your team, it is important to make those expectations known. It will never be possible to create enough documents to address every situation that may come up or go wrong in a research project. Thus, you want to establish a culture and work environment so that your staff know the *processes* to solve problems and communicate with others. Consider an emphasis on your team or lab's values, culture, and processes rather than trying to list rules to fit every situation.

Meaningful Moments

Teams function optimally when they understand their objectives, when roles are clear, and when individual team members are both respected for their contribution(s) and trusted to do what is required. Therefore, I begin all relationships with each member of my team by creating a mentoring agreement that allows us to align our expectations of one another, describe how we will maintain effective communications, and how I will assess their understanding, identify the causes of any lack of understanding, and create strategies to address misunderstanding.

— Beth Meyerand, PhD

We all know that planning a research project involves drawing up documents that plan the project and its ideas. Similarly, a few key documents are needed to represent your team or lab culture and key processes. We suggest the following documents become part of your team or lab's work. Further, we suggest these documents should be rooted in your vision and mission for your research that you developed in Chap. 2. In many cases you may not need to develop all of these documents anew, as your colleagues may have versions of their own that you could review and ask to use as starting points.

Documents to build for your team:

1. *Team culture and values document*: In this document, you explain your lab/team's culture. Is your team meant to be ambitious, cutting edge, and hierarchical with opportunities to move up? Is your team meant to be collaborative, sharing, and structured using a UN model? There is no right or wrong answer, but writing up your vision can help your team understand what you expect and help potential new team members determine if they can function well in that team culture.

2. *Statement of professional ethics*: In this document you outline clear expectations around research lab ethics. These expectations are best situated within your team culture and values. This document typically outlines for and reminds team members of critical behaviors that are not tolerated. For example, falsification of data, or sharing information at a party about a research participant's behavior. These lab ethics should link to the values you hold on your team, such as data integrity and respect for participants.
3. *Policies and procedures*: It is likely that your institution has a policy document, or even an honor code, so be sure to include these in your orientations for your team members. If you have specific policies you want to have on everyone's radar, draw up your own adjunct policy document. For example, if there are critical times of the year for your project where staff cannot take vacation time, spell those out so everyone knows this in advance.

Developing Your Own Manager Skills

Being the PI of a research lab or team is a tricky task. It involves expertise across several roles, roles that in many places such as the business world, are often represented by separate people. You are first and foremost the generator of new ideas and visions for your science. So, you are the CEO. You are also in charge of building your team and getting the best people to help you to rock your science. So, you are also the director of HR. You also need to establish how work will flow, and how individual research projects will be organized to achieve deadlines. This means you are also a project manager.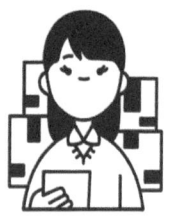

For many scientists, the organizational and managerial aspects of running their lab are tasks they exasperatedly describe as "not something I was trained for." However, investing a small amount of time and energy in your skills and knowledge can have big payoff. We recommend taking some time to review your reflections from Chap. 2 and to consider your strengths and areas you are still developing. We have included a resource list at the end of the book if you would like some recommendations for additional ways to approach these important areas of your work.

Your Colleagues

Nurturing colleagues is a fruitful way to both enhance your career and your life. For these types of relationships, areas of research or topic interest may be less important, as the focus is on people you like to talk with and get along with and can make time for each other. Often these relationships emerge naturally, your desks are near each other at work and you find that you get along. You completed training around the same time, or your kids are about the same age. It often does not take effort to find these folks, but the critical skill and effort are to maintain them over time.

Why take the time to maintain these relationships? Engaging with colleagues can lead to enhanced productivity as well as joy. You can get new ideas and critical feedback. These are often the people you can talk with about a political drama at work, or your disappointment in not getting a grant you really wanted, because they are your colleagues and not your supervisors. You can talk about organization, as well as the management and structure of your research teams, learning from each other.

At its most basic level, taking time with colleagues to laugh, celebrate, brainstorm or cry is a form of self-care.

Ways to nurture your relationships with colleagues: Put a recurring reminder on your calendar for every 3–4 months to check in with your colleague. Meet for happy hour, do a walking meeting, or just work together at the same coffee shop. If you both have grant deadlines coming up, and you need to work a weekend day, consider meeting at the lab at the same time to work, and schedule a coffee break midway through the day to encourage each other.

Your Close Collaborators

Another source of joy, inspiration, and productivity in your inner circle are your close collaborators. In the early stages of your career, you likely will be focused on developing mentorship relationships and close colleagues. Over time, you will develop a network of collaborators, and it is never too early to consider how you will approach this and what type of collaborators you hope to find.

Your close collaborators will include people you consider co-investigators, on your grants, your papers, and your projects. They bring valuable expertise to your work, allowing your work to have a more expansive scope while keeping your own research focus laser-sharp and focused. Some of them may become colleagues or even work-friends.

A key aspect of seeking collaborators is to bring diversity to your work. This means diversity in people and the richness that diversity brings to your team. Diversity in training, expertise, background, seniority in career stage, race/ethnicity, gender, and culture are among the valued ways that you can seek diverse collaborators. This also means diversity in expertise, which may include seeking out people with expertise in different research methods, topic areas, or analysis techniques. In some cases, your collaborators may include people with expertise beyond research, such as programmers or communication specialists.

Meaningful Moments
Finding lasting solutions to address health disparities requires creativity, flexibility, and tenacity. We are continually designing, testing, refining, and evaluating interventions; cycling through Plan A, B, C and D in the pursuit of our research objectives. We strategize and brainstorm—Daily. With the aim to promote adolescent health, we work closely with designers, programmers, and videographers to craft compelling content, grounded in behavior-change theory, and use Design Thinking methods to align our interventions to the needs of the target audience.

—Stephanie Craig Rushing, PhD, MPH

Your Mentees

We have book-ended this chapter with ideas about mentoring. In the first part, we discussed finding and evaluating your own mentors. We now turn our attention to your role as a mentor. Just as you consider the values and skills you seek in a mentor, you must consider what values and skills you represent to others.

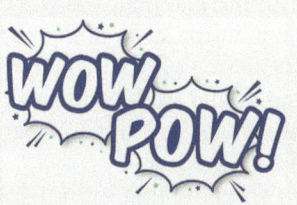

Katya was a junior faculty just starting work on her career development grant. She was approached by an undergraduate student in nursing named Mary who was interested in having a research experience. Mary had no previous research experience, but she was considering getting her PhD in nursing and wanted to have a lab experience to be sure. Mary was willing to work as a volunteer. Katya invited Mary to join her team as an undergraduate research intern, and Mary was reliable and a good contributor to Katya's projects. After a few months Mary asked if she could do her own independent analyses of some extra data, on her own time. Katya was surprised but excited to provide support and mentorship. Mary presented her project at the undergraduate research symposium, and then asked to do a summer internship to include writing up her project as a paper. Again surprised, Katya reasoned it would be good practice for her to help coach someone through writing a paper. Mary completed the paper and was published in a peer-reviewed journal with Katya as senior author. A few years later, Katya received a mentoring award and learned that Mary had written a very strong letter on her behalf. Based on these experiences, Katya developed systems to include undergraduates in her lab and offer them presenting and writing experiences.

Another myth to bust is that you need to wait to have gray hair before mentoring. The reality is you can mentor as soon as have made a commitment to doing so and some information or skills to share. Maybe you have done your first research project as a PhD student and now you are a post doc; an undergraduate seeks you out for mentorship on a class project. You can be a mentor.

It is important to know that even if you are early in your career, there are immense benefits to being a mentor. There are also some risks.

The benefits are that you are likely to become a better mentee by having experience on both sides of the equation. You are likely to become a better scientist if you are teaching what you practice. You may get new ideas from engaging with your mentee, and you may even be more productive if your mentee is presenting or publishing work with you as the senior author.

However, all these benefits are null and void if you spend so much time on your mentee that you are not able to do your own science. You may get too focused on a mentee, particularly on trying to fix an unproductive one. Remember being a mentor is an altruistic role. You do it to help guide and support a person. But you do not do it to correct a meandering rudderless boat with no captain on board. Your own science will suffer. You will not be able to get a grant funded without writing it. You will not get a paper published without completing the experiments. You will not get a job by explaining that you focused so much time on your mentees you were unable to achieve anything of your own.

What to do with the rudderless boat? Well, you have a few options. One is to call in a second opinion, ask the mentee to set up some meetings with other potential mentors. It may be that there is a style mismatch that another mentor could overcome and bring out a purpose or vision for that mentee, or take on the role of primary mentor if the style match is better. Another option is to be transparent and direct with the mentee, to let them know the challenges you are facing in your role as mentor. You can consider giving the person a time frame by which they need to have a plan of action, and/or let them know you need to step back from being a primary mentor but can remain a big picture mentor.

What to do with the needy mentee? Again, you have options. One is to seek input from your own mentors. It may be possible to ask a more senior member of your research team or lab (a graduate student for example) to help co-mentor a student needing additional support. Providing mentees more than one mentor provides them the same multi-mentor support we have recommended for your career.

What to do with a mentee who is struggling? Struggling could include performance concerns, or even just issues with showing up consistently or on time. This is definitely a scenario in which you would want to seek other input and expertise. You will benefit from input from your mentors and may even include other institutional supports. For example, if the mentee is a student, you may want to see if student services can help. This is particularly of benefit if you think that there may be aspects of the mentee's life that are interfering with their work. We know that many students are dealing with academic, financial, and life stressors, so their struggle may represent something that goes beyond your lab. That doesn't mean it is your problem to fix, but being kind and connecting them to resources may go a long way for a future scientist.

Overall, we hope that the take-home here is that balance is the key. We would have more women rocking science if more of us mentored earlier and supported early career scientists. However, mentoring comes with risks that need to be evaluated early and often.

If you choose to mentor, screening potential mentees is important. Mentees that want to take on a project "to look good on my resume" or "to get into medical school" are probably higher risk. Mentees who want experience doing a project, or who are interested in your area of work, or who are unsure about their future and curious about science, are likely to be more invested in finishing their work. Use the informational interview to your advantage as a mentor. We will discuss this more in Chap. 7.

Take-Home Points

Your innermost circle of your SEM is critical to your productivity and success.

Take time to consider your needs, strengths, and opportunities.

Schedule time for this reflection for yourself on a regular basis.

Invest in cultivating your mentors, your team members, your colleagues, and your own mentees.

Homework
- Map out your process for identifying, evaluating, and maintaining mentors.
- Develop a plan for your research team size, structure, culture, and key expectations.
- Create a plan to nurture your relationships with colleagues.
- Consider your own strengths and skills you can offer a mentee.

.

Chapter 4
Your Institutional Support/Academic Environment

Institutional support is paramount for faculty advancement. There are multitudes of ways your institution is built to help you. In this chapter we will describe the second circle in the socioecological model (described in Chap. 1), your institution, and how the support of your institution is fundamental to your development as a researcher and scientist as well as to the development of your team. Although identifying what your institutional support is may feel like hide-and-seek, really this is seek-and-find. There is a lot out there; you just have to intentionally and purposefully look for it all.

What Is Your "Institution"?

A simplistic description of your institution is that it is the organization that hired you. In many cases in academic clinical research, your institution is your university. Your institution is not that simple though; it is, in fact, quite complex. Within your specific institution, there are multiple levels or organization within it. Key players for you may include your boss(es), your research unit, your clinical division or section, and your department. At some institutions, the clinical enterprise may be a separate but connected entity; in others, it is all one organization. At a college or university, your institu-

M. A. Moreno, R. Katzenellenbogen, *Women Rock Science*, https://doi.org/10.1007/978-3-031-48418-6_4

tion is also your school within that university, the university as a whole, and even a large university's multi-campus locations. Therefore, your institution is a single entity. But it has many different layers to it—much like your career or, dare we say it, a socioecological model.

What *Does* Your Institution Offer to You?

You are an important component of any institution. Without you and your colleagues, your institution is merely empty buildings with echoing hallways. As a means of supporting you, your institution has innate characteristics and facilities built within it to support your career goals and specifically your research goals. Those characteristics and facilities should be in place the day you walk in, and you need to know what your institution is ready to do for you the moment you arrive, so you can rock your science.

Your institution has *libraries*. These house books, journals, and source materials in real buildings! Increasingly, libraries also function electronically with institutional subscriptions to electronically accessible books and journals. Libraries are still run by librarians—real people—and they are a wealth of information on how to execute literature searches, how to find and source data, and how to dig through old stacks for historic materials.

Real-time advice: Most libraries have a designated librarian assigned to different departments. Take the time to go there and meet the librarian assigned to your department. You can treat this meeting like an informational interview (as described in Chap. 3); learn their interests and share yours. Find out her recommendations for the best ways you can work with her when you need help with things like a literature review for a new grant, or a potential systematic review paper on your research topic. Then when you need help with those activities, you already know a person to contact (and potentially a new friendly colleague as a bonus).

Some libraries also offer trainings in tools you may use for research. These include reference management programs to electronically store and document your empirical citations for your manuscripts. These trainings will be useful to you, as well as potentially useful for your team or to recommend to your colleagues and mentees.

Your institution also has *stuff*—lots and lots of stuff. Copiers, scanners, paper, folders, even pens and pencils are all items that your institution has in order to support you and your research. Your institution should provide you access to work space including a desk, bookshelves and file cabinets, a telephone, and outlets. It is the case that some institutions have developed different space regulations and shifts in resources since the COVID-19 pandemic. With many institutions adopting more flexible work location policies, some have reduced available office space with expanded use and support of software programs and digital applications to facilitate virtual and hybrid work. This is something to look into with any new position.

Your institution should also provide you a computer and other hardware, internet access, software applications, network drives, and back up storage for the data, manuscripts, grants, and clinical work you generate. It should provide opportunities to elevate and promote your work, such as through websites about you and your research, promoting the innovative work being done at your institution. Invariably, all of these things will break down or experience hiccups, and your institution has IT, building, and engineering staff in place to help fix them all. Most of these materials, people, or expenses are not drawn from your budget or salary—they are costs of doing business and being an institution. Some of these costs are covered through indirect costs on grants across your department, your school, or your campus.

Your institution has *core facilities* for research. These facilities are typically run by research scientists who themselves may not develop and execute novel research projects. Rather, they support the work of independent principal investigators with their rich technical knowledge on a specific topic or methodology, and they often run dedicated pieces of (expensive) equipment. These core facilities can include histopathology, antibody development, flow cytometry, genomics, biostatistics, specimen storage, animal care/housing, phlebotomy/lab, and scientific imaging. They are often discounted (or even free!) for those who are members of the institution, are available to researchers who budget for them on grants, or are available on a fee-for-service basis. Whatever their role, core facilities, and the people who run them are key to the success of most researchers. Without them, you will literally be reinventing the wheel!

Real-time advice: If you do not know the range of core facilities at your institution, take some time to explore these. You never know what new idea will arise when you realize you could combine a known technique with something new you did not know you could do. Get to know the staff that work in these facilities and show them kindness and respect. It is helpful to develop your own network (as part of your SEM!) on campus, and you may find yourself needing a last minute favor from them sometime.

Most institutions support core facilities, but all institutions have *shared equipment*. This is because scientific equipment is very expensive. In order to justify their utility, their purchase comes with a mandate for researchers to share them. These can include confocal microscopes, ultracentrifuges, freezers, mass spectrometry, HPLC machines, biosafety cabinets and fume hoods, bacterial shakers, and real-time PCR machines. Some shared equipment falls under the umbrella of core facilities, but many of these pieces of equipment are housed within a specific lab or research group and do not require direct oversight by a research scientist.

Real-time advice: If your projects rely on shared equipment, get to know the others with whom who you will be sharing. Developing a collegial relationship early, and understanding key deadlines or timelines for them and for you, will help you ensure you can get your projects done on time.

Institutions have *shared oversight* to support the research they conduct. These are often mandated by codes, laws, and guidelines, but institutions can execute these in different ways. All institutions that conduct research involving animals or human subjects have animal care offices, IACUC, and IRBs. They also all have environmental health and safety offices to assure hazardous materials are handled appropriately and safely. Institutions also have offices dedicated to the submission and management of your grants. There are Sponsored Project Offices that accurately submit your grant applications and manage your budgets, along with department and research administrators who help facilitate the work that goes into these products.

Real-time advice: Get to know the people in these offices and positions. Set up an appointment and go there in person, notebook (electronic or paper) in hand. All institutions and funding agencies have specific rules and guidelines that need to be followed, and you want to know what those are. For example, your institution's Offices for Research Grants might require all grants to be submitted for institutional approvals at least 7 days before the funding agency's grant deadline. This is something you want to know waaaaay before submitting your first grant so you can plan your timeline accordingly. Further, these folks often have depth of knowledge and experience in grant submissions, you can learn a great deal from them if you ask.

Finally, your institution has *administrative support*. Office staff, program coordinators, security officers, custodial staff, commuter services, and grounds keepers all keep your institution working. Without them, nothing gets done!

Real-time advice: Administrative support people are the folks who get things done at your institution, but they do not always receive the respect they deserve. You have the opportunity to be a faculty member who gives respect across all levels of your institution. Not only is this good strategy when it comes time to ask for help from people in administrative roles, but it is just part of being a good human.

Meaningful Moments
My first faculty position out of fellowship as a junior faculty researcher was at a smaller institution which did not have the infrastructure in place to facilitate clinical or translational research. I felt very much alone in my search for support with sample acquisition, processing and storage, information regarding hiring lab staff, freezer monitoring, etc. I learned the processes and systems on my own by trial and error. In retrospect, I should have asked more questions about the research infrastructure in place prior to accepting a faculty position.
  — Terri Laguna, MD

What *Should* Your Institution Offer to You?

So, as you can see, your institution has a lot of people and things that are ready to help you and your research. Some are tangible, and some are abstract. However, your institution also should offer you items required to get a running start on your research. This is true whether your science is at its beginning, or you have been rocking it for years. Every scientist has unique needs to get her work done. Because of that, your institution should give you *start-up funds* or a *start-up package*. These may include a single or multiple sources of funds, or line item expenses and support for those. These funds are typically used for equipment, software, reagents, materials, technology, and personnel that you will need to begin or resume your work, or a package may include those items. Funds can sometimes be used to protect your time for research — allowing you to focus on your research and scientific development without the need to find grants to cover your time — but this is often negotiated separately at the time of hire or when you get new grants. Some institutions ask for a line item proposed budget, others offer a lump sum and leave to you to determine its use. Like a quart of milk....be sure to pay attention to expiration dates!

Real-time advice: Start-up funds vary by institution, by research type and needs, and by the individual. Ask colleagues or mentors to provide strategies and ideas for what could be included in your start-up funds. A near-peer mentor who recently went through this process could be an invaluable source of what the current landscape is on these types of packages. Be reasonable, but do not be shy—ask for what you need. An institution will rarely tell you that you did not ask for enough (they are happy to "get a deal") and things often cost more or take more time than you expect! Getting input from others will help you understand whether what you are being offered is reasonable, for your type of science.

Institutions also should have funds for *pilot projects* or a *pilot grant program*. These are projects based on ideas, hypothesis-driven, that need data in order to be established as valid. They are funds for small, short projects that will leapfrog an idea to creation of foundational data for a grant. Pilot funding may be at the university level, school level, or even within your department or research center.

Real-time advice: Find out the deadlines for pilot grant funding, and put them on your calendar so you can plan ahead for these. There is often much less competition for these grants compared to national competition for federal funds. Early-stage investigators are often prioritized in these grant competitions, so you want to optimize the timing of your own application.

Institutions should also have *bridge funds*. These are funds that support a researcher during gaps in extramural (outside) funding, so her projects can continue, data can be generated, research teams can remain cohesive and intact, and study participants can be retained. This approach helps laboratories and research teams avoid shutting down and then having to restart based solely on the capricious nature of federal and philanthropic funding agencies.

Real-time advice: Know your institution's policies on bridge funds and before you ever anticipate needing them.

Work closely with your financial grants managers to monitor your spending. Strategically plan the timing of grant proposals to mitigate the need for bridge funding.

To expand your ideas and skillsets, institutions should also support your *career development*. This support can come in many forms. Professional development programs internal and external to your institution will help you become a well-rounded scientist and academician. Financial support for continuing education courses, executive management, license fees, maintenance of certification, and travel to conferences are all critical to your work, your success, and your career. Periodic sabbaticals are established for a researcher to learn new skills from colleagues around the world.

Real-time advice: Keep track of your career development ideas and needs within your lab notebook or another saved document (perhaps in the folder with your individual academic development plan and mission statement you developed in Chap. 2). If there is a resource you need, use the document to build the idea. Note experiences in which that career development need arose and how you could have leveraged that resource. Then, when the time comes to make the ask of your institution for additional resources, you have a thoughtful plan and supporting evidence already in motion.

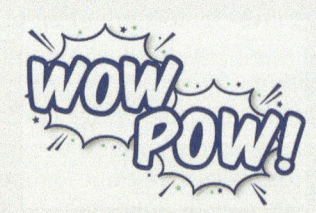

Nikita is a recently hired junior faculty. Before she arrives, the division head who recruited her takes a position at another academic institution. She now has an interim head who is only there to "keep the ship pointed straight." There is so much disruption in the division with the loss of this leader that she cannot even get on her interim division head's calendar. She tries to contact her department chair, but she is out of the country. How to solve this? Some parts of this situation are clearly not in Nikita's realm to solve. But to navigate this situation, she still needs to work on seeking support, advice, guidance and resources. She reaches out to mid-career faculty in her division and sets up meetings to understand how to navigate division resources (and politics). Through these meetings, she hears about some supportive mentors in another division, as well as contacts in a different division who recently experienced this. She even hears about a newer faculty in a different department with similar interests to hers. She sets up meetings with these people and gets ideas, support and connections to others in her department and beyond.

Career development also can meld into the realm of equity and work–life balance. Faculty development programs recognize people strengths and opportunities for their career advancement. Time management courses. Mindfulness sessions. Leadership and communication workshops. Without a solid foundation of wellness, appreciation of diversity, and a good balance of time, careers collapse.

Career development also means ensuring that institutions promote *diversity in science*. For faculty members of color, from underrepresented minority groups, from different cultures, with different physical or mental abilities, or from the LGBTQI+ community, it is important to identify what specific groups or resources are available at your institution. These may include a diversity task force, disability resources, a council for same-gender faculty members, committees to support faculty members of color, or leadership positions focused on diversity, equity, inclusivity, and accessibility. Find your community within the institution (or create one!), and meet with leadership that supports your needs. This can be an important source of professional and personal support, and garner access to specific programs to accelerate your work.

In addition to being supported as a faculty member by task forces and resources that focus on diversity in science, you could consider joining these as a member yourself. As women in science, you come to your work with a different lens. Your voice is important. If you identify as a gender minority and a racial or ethnic minority, you represent an intersectionality has unique perspectives and strengths. And you have the opportunity to bring more than one perspective to any discussion. We recognize that there is a minority tax on people who are asked, again and again, to represent a group that is not the majority. However, this is also a chance to create change for the better. It may feel valuable to you to join in when an opportunity aligns with your interests and identity.

For any faculty member, even with good planning and practice, roadblocks and obstacles come up. Institutions should have benefit programs to meet those needs. Bereavement, medical leave, family leave, daycare and sick daycare access, and mental health counseling are all examples. These resources are ones you may not ever plan on needing. They are essential supports, however, when life events happen, expected or not, helping to keep you on track in your own career path.

Finally, your institution has a *tenure system*. Tenure was established to protect your intellectual pursuits from the vagaries of funding and the whim of people in power. Once promoted to a tenured position, you cannot be terminated because your research or teachings go against the leanings of others. Achieving tenure also implies that your career path has been seen as valuable and productive by your peers across the country. Your institution rewards you with job protection and a big feather in your cap. Some institutions have guaranteed salary support along with a tenured position.

Others simply guarantee your position but require you still to support your salary directly by your work—be it teaching, research, clinical care, or administrative work. We will discuss the promotion process, and its requirements, in Chap. 6.

How Does Your Institution Assure Their Faculty Advance?

Mentoring! *Mentors* help guide your career from start to finish. They may play a role in one component of your career or they may guide all of it. Chapter 3 covers information about how to identify your mentoring needs, and seek out and evaluate potential mentors.

> **Meaningful Moments**
> I was lucky that I started my independent position on the same day as another Assistant Professor in my department, so I had someone to navigate through the maze of institutional support and resources with me. However, I also sought the advice of someone who was still junior faculty but had started a few years before me and knew the ropes. In addition, I had a great department chair that was very accessible and willing to answer any questions.
> —Cary Moody, PhD

In many institutions, you will have a *mentoring committee* who oversees your development, and they collectively shepherd you through your academic work toward the goal of being promoted in rank from Assistant Professor to Associate Professor or the like. Mentors can come from your home division or department. They also can come from other segments of your institution, especially if they bring a unique expertise you will need to meet your goals.

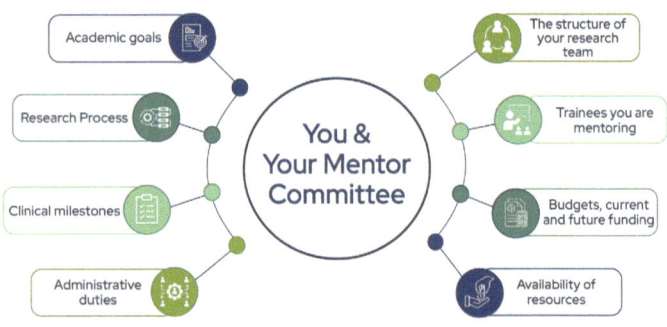

FIGURE 4.1 You and your mentor committee: Possible discussion topics and area of work

Whoever they are, your mentor committee should meet with you at established times to review your (Fig. 4.1):

Before these meetings, you should review your individual academic development plan and your mission statement (Chap. 2). These will center your meeting's purpose.

Real-time advice: Your institution should help facilitate your mentoring committee using a formalized structure. This is something to ask about. How are your mentors chosen? Are they assigned? Do you find them yourselves? Do you document and take minutes at your meetings with your mentor or mentoring committee? How are they logged? How often are you expected to meet and review your goals and your progress? What do you do if a mentor, or your committee, is unhelpful? At the start of your career, meetings with your committee should happen on a semiannual or quarterly basis. Once more established, you can meet with your mentor committee formally once a year, and as needed. Some institutions have rules around mentor committee meeting frequency, be sure to know what those are to meet your promotion milestones and requirements.

In additional to your mentor or mentors, you will have an *annual review*. Your section, division, or department heads should meet with you regularly and confirm you are reaching critical milestones on your promotion pathway.

Keep in mind: Mentors coach you. They give you advice based on their own expertise. They may have a bias in their recommendations, but those can be balanced by other members of a committee. Your division or department head also coaches you, but her role is also to evaluate you. Your bosses mark your level of achievement and will sing your praises, or will wave red warning flags, as you move toward and through promotion.

Where Do You Find Your Institution's Resources?

This is a daunting question. It is more than what is listed on the Human Resources page. Parts of this need to be negotiated as a part of your job description and recruitment package. Institutional support can come from your home division or department, but it also can span colleagues, departments, and centers, if you develop shared cross-disciplinary research or clinical practices.

Lessons from the Lab

I chose to join the faculty where I (Rachel) had trained after medical school. As a trainee, you know everything about where you work—the phone numbers for every office, where every bathroom is, and who is helpful when you need it. Yet, you also know almost nothing about the infrastructure and resources available to you as faculty when you are a trainee. I went to new faculty orientation when I was formally hired on the tenure track, 10 years after I had come to the university to train, and it was eye-opening. There were areas of campus I had never even walked to! With that, I also came to realize that the institution around me was not static. Presidents of the university came and went. Focus and mandates were developed, implemented, and scrapped. I paid attention to these changes and movements, and jumped on those that were fun and exciting to consider. Despite staying in the same place for many years as a trainee and faculty member, my roles and needs changed over time. Think about how yours may as well.

So, how do you do it? How do you find these resources?

Ask.
Ask again.
Ask everyone.

It is the responsibility of your bosses to tell you what is available. It is the goal of your mentors to help you find these resources and to point you in the right direction. Your mentors need to know you and make sure your institution works best for you. However, at this point in anyone's career, you will need to do some footwork on your own. No one is going to spoon feed you. You are now a scientist, a specialist in your academic career. You are unique—your needs are not mirrored in anyone else's career. It's time to "take the bull by the horns." Self-advocacy and personal motivation are critical to leveraging all of the resources your institution has in place, so you achieve your maximal growth.

What do you do if your division head does nothing for you? Laissez-faire at its best…negligent at its worst… What do you do if you are on your own?

How do you leverage support for your needs if that person is not "really in charge?"

How do you know what you even need because you are just so new?

This is when footwork is critical. Begin to develop your own network of people and resources yourself. Review websites from Human Resources and beyond. Benefits pages. Commuter and transportation tools. Faculty Development Offices and programming. Department and division pages and faculty directories. Email people, set up in-person meetings to meet face-to-face and introduce yourself. Bring a synopsis of who you are and what you plan to do. This is where a mission statement is valuable (Chap. 2). Let that person describe their work and determine where your expertise and interests may overlap and could be synergistic. Spend real time establishing this network at the start of your career at a new institution. Understanding your institution's landscape will allow you to know who to call when you need something for a critical project. Consider including in your recruitment and start-up package protected time to hold these meetings and research your needed resources. This will ultimately allow you to "mentor up" and guide your mentor(s) through what you really need and what you really want.

Meaningful Moments
The best way to learn about these is to network with other senior faculty, junior faculty, and trainees, in as many venues as feasible—interacting with those who have backgrounds different from your own will often provide a different perspective and awareness of different institutional resources. Even for me, it is not uncommon that it is precisely the seminar that I think has very little relevance to my own work, which ends up providing me with new ideas, new connections, and new collaborations.
—Ursula Kaiser, MD

What is critical to remember is this: your institution surrounds you in your career development and advancement. Your institution should work to identify barriers and remove them wholly on your behalf. It should nominate you for opportunities that will support your career. It should protect you from opportunities that will stagnate your career.

What Is Your Academic Environment? How Is That Different Than Your Institution?

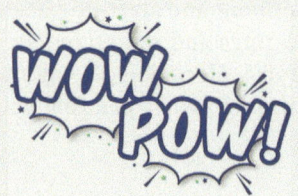

Toni-Ann goes to a seminar where a colleague at a department across campus is presenting. She is using new analytic software that Toni-Ann read about in a recent journal article, and her group's findings are fantastic. After the seminar, she greets the speaker, complements her on this work and asks about the software. She offers for Toni-Ann to come to her office to discuss her project and the software next week and will arrange to have her research associate there to demonstrate how to use it in case she would like to trial it with her own data.

Whereas your institution represents the structure and personnel that make up your work environment, your academic environment is different. It is broader than your institution. It is the feeling, the ethos, the energy of your institution.

What does your institution care about? The answer lies within your academic environment (Fig. 4.2).The academic environment is as important as the institutional structure is. The academic environment can be energizing, combative, or toxic.

FIGURE 4.2 Examples of priorities for academic medical institutions

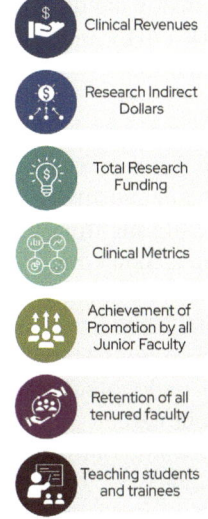

Clinical Revenues

Research Indirect Dollars

Total Research Funding

Clinical Metrics

Achievement of Promotion by all Junior Faculty

Retention of all tenured faculty

Teaching students and trainees

Meaningful Moments
Institutions vary greatly in their expectations for faculty, and their tolerance and support for work/life balance as well. If possible, interview current junior faculty about their experiences to see if the environment is a "good fit." Your "preparation" for selecting the best environment for your faculty career should include understanding not only the resources, but the climate of your potential professional home.
— Yolanda (Linda) Reid Chassiokas, MD

The academic environment of an institution can vary across departments. What is collegial in one is back-stabbing in another. Luckily, the academic environment can be changed with good leadership, but that can take time. When you consider a new position in academic science, ask about this issue. Pay attention to people's responses. Are they hesitant? Effusive? Wavering? You will not be able to find this out on any website or in any handbook. You will only determine the ethos of a work environment and institution by your own personal investigation.

Take-Home Points

There are many resources and supports in academic institutions, and the academic environments flavor that support.

Your bosses and mentors will help you find institutional support, but you also need to look for them yourself. You are an independent researcher and scientist. You identify and study new questions yourself, so trust you are good at this! The relationships you develop in learning about these types of support will undoubtedly pay off, in the short term and long term, in your career.

Determining what your institution has available is not just other people's jobs.

It is a critical part of your job. Dig deep. Ask. Listen. Act.

If you do not, the only person you are hindering is yourself.

Homework

- Identify your bosses and where they fall in scope and rank.
- Identify resources you need to do your work: Think about your workday from start to finish and all institutional supports that may be involved. Then go meet with each of the people involved in that support.
- Identify resources you need to balance work within your life.
- Set up a calendar for required tasks on your promotion track:
  - Meet with the promotion administrators to align your CV style and other reporting documents with what you'll need for promotion.
  - Consider if you can leverage administrative support to have ongoing scheduled updates of your CV.
- Leverage the academic development plan that you created in Chap. 2 to structure your mentor meetings and note achievements gained.

Chapter 5
Your Scientific Community

In this chapter we want to start a conversation about growing beyond your home turf. You do your science locally; it takes place within your team at your institution. But also, you are also a scientist within a **larger global scientific community** — a community full of peers, colleagues, and people with similar or related purpose and goal. Within this larger community, you contribute new knowledge to advance a field of work. Thus, it is important to consider ways you connect to that larger scientific community. We will address several areas of this larger scientific community in this chapter. First, we will consider professional societies that provide academic stimulation and collaboration. Second, we will address contributing to science's big picture, including reviewing grants and papers, and attending conferences. Finally, we invite you to consider your role among your own circle of learners, either geographical or topical, and ways to contribute to the future of science.

© The Author(s), under exclusive license to Springer Nature
Switzerland AG 2024
M. A. Moreno, R. Katzenellenbogen, *Women Rock Science*,
https://doi.org/10.1007/978-3-031-48418-6_5

This level of engagement with the larger scientific community is the furthest circle in your socioecological model. This type of engagement is often the one that junior scientists first defer, focusing instead on mastering their own research mission and understanding their immediate environments. However, as women and gender diverse scientists in particular, there are reasons to look to this larger community early in your career. Literature suggests that women leaders are uniquely skilled at building networks and relationships in their work and derive benefit in their own work from these efforts. Women and gender diverse scientists often feel a strong sense of purpose by seeing their work reflected in a larger community and by building bridges into the scientific community to understand current research trends and issues. Having connections to this community can protect a scientist from a feeling of isolation that can impede a research career, and the research itself, at certain stages. Considering the level of the individual scientist, reaching into the larger scientific community can provide passion for one's work by seeing the bigger picture, or the larger potential benefit, of one's work (Fig. 5.1).

FIGURE 5.1 Scientific community

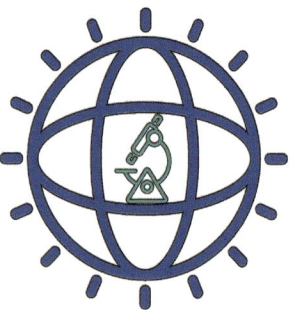

Joining Professional Societies

Professional societies are organizations that provide membership and community to professionals who work in a particular topic area. They have a mission statement, a focus, and a purpose. For academic clinical researchers, these professional organizations may be clinical, disease-focused, or research-focused. Table 5.1 lists some categories of professional societies that academic clinical researchers may join in their career journey.

While the specific focus of a professional society may vary, their overall mission is often to provide *education, information distribution, and a shared community*. These organizations provide several functions within their scope of work. These functions may include publishing academic journals, organizing conferences to present the latest research, promoting policies or practice standards, and giving awards to members. Because these organizations are typically not beholden to a particular university, federal agency, political party or agenda, they typically have a high degree of credibility and influence in the field. These professional organizations are often looked to as a source to define and set standards for their respective fields.

What Can You Get out of a Professional Society?

Meaningful Moments
Don't take your alma mater or other early professional relationships for granted; they can impact your future in positive ways that you might not initially foresee.
—Heidi Wagner, OD.

Similar interests: A professional society can offer you the opportunity to engage with others in your field who share similar interests. These are "your people." Societies often draw members from all levels within a profession,

TABLE 5.1 Examples of professional societies

Types of professional societies	Examples
Clinical practice focused	American Medical Association, American Academy of Pediatrics
Clinical and research focused	Society for Adolescent Health and Medicine, Pediatric Endocrine Society, American Association for Cancer Research, American Society for Microbiology, Pediatric Infectious Disease Society
Research topic/type focus	Society for Research in Child Development, Society for Behavioral Medicine, International Society of Virology, International Papillomavirus Society
Research field focus	Society for Pediatric Research, American Pediatric Society, Academic Pediatric Association
Research method focus	Statistical Society, International Internet Interventions Research Society
Academic or research interest groups	Societies focused on specific groups in science or medicine (e.g. gender, LGBTQI+, culture, geography), Graduate Women in Medicine and Science, Well-being focused groups

from trainees to emeritus professors. If you happen to be at a university where there are few colleagues with similar work to yours, a society is a way to build yourself a research community of people who share your interests and passions.

Cognitive diversity: While your professional society can offer you like-minded peers, it can also be a source of cognitive diversity. You may find peers with similar interests, but differences in communication styles, problem solving, writing strategy, or experimental designs. This can lead to new ideas and collaborations and richer creativity.

New mentors: You may find new mentors at a professional society. Finding mentors within your professional society may be of particular interest to you if there are no mentors at your home institution in your particular research niche.

Connections for promotion: As you plan ahead to rock your promotion (more on this in Chap. 6), you will need to plan for external letters of reference. Your professional society is a place in which you can identify those faculty who could serve as an external letter of reference.

Your professional home: For most researchers, finding a primary "home" organization is important. It provides you benefits to engage with an organization over the long term to enrich your research productivity and ideas, and your identity as a scientist among your peers. It can provide you long-term relationships that can provide joy and enrichment during downturns in your research or productivity. As you probably know, over the course of your career, you and your peers may change institutions. Your professional home can be a way to keep in touch and have a place to be together each year at the organization's conference.

See the big picture: One benefit of membership within professional societies is that these organizations may have a clearer overview of trends in their fields than federal agencies, universities, and funding organizations. It is the place you can get the inside scoop. Understanding trends in new research findings presented at a yearly conference can give you unique insight on what areas of research are likely to be growing in the very near future, and what areas are already played out.

How to Pick Your Professional Society

An ideal professional society will provide you several things:

1. A yearly meeting to attend (see next section on how to best use these meetings).

(a) Opportunities to submit your research for peer-review in order to present at that meeting.

(b) Opportunities to view others' research, and meet peers and potential collaborators with similar work.

(c) Workshops or sessions to enrich your knowledge base, or gain new academic skills. An example academic workshop may be on grant writing or leadership skills. You may also consider seeking out workshops or sessions focused on women or gender diversity in science.

(d) Opportunities to meet with and socialize with old and new friends, peers, mentors, collaborators, and colleagues.

(e) Connections to others in your field at various levels of seniority.

(f) Have reduced registration fees as an active member.

2. Opportunities to submit your research for peer-review to an academic journal.

(a) Have reduced publication costs as an active member.

3. Opportunities to participate in committees with a focus on a specific subtopic.

4. Opportunities for leadership within the organization.

5. Opportunities to draft position statements or review articles on topics in research and academics.

Why Would You *Not* Join a Professional Society?

Cost: This can be a barrier for sure. Some professional societies have costs that seem out of proportion to their value. Most societies do have reduced rates for trainees or early faculty. Ideally, your institution should provide support for you to join professional societies. It can only benefit them to have you representing your institution at a national or international organizational level. If institutional support to join your professional society is lacking, you can advocate for the benefits that your institute will gain with your membership. These benefits may include presenting at the society's national meeting (with your gorgeous poster with the institution's logo on it), or a national committee membership that brings recognition to your institution.

I have so much to do: You do have a lot to do! If we revisit your socioecological framework, you have your individual work and research to attend to, your team to manage and care for, and your institution to please. Your professional society forms that next circle out in your socioecological model. Without this layer of your socioecological model, you are missing a valuable source of new research ideas to inform your work, information and strategy that can optimize your team's function, and chances for national recognition that can make or break your promotion. We recommend considering the cost of NOT doing this important work.

What Can You **Do** in a Professional Society?

Sign up: A first step is to join the society. Membership may include a journal subscription or being on a listserv. Listservs, ugh, we know. It can be helpful to keep an eye on the listserv early in your membership to understand a little about the culture of the organization, but by no means do you need to read every email.

Go: If the society has a yearly conference, start attending. If this society is going to be your "professional home," it is a good idea to begin a track record of attending. More information about going to conferences is below.

Join a committee: If the society has committees, look over the list and see if any are of interest. If a committee is of interest, approach a committee member or the leaders to express interest and ask about what is involved in joining. In general, *most* committee memberships do not require a lot of time or work at the professional society level. For real. Often it includes attending that committee's meeting during the yearly conference, or work that comes once a year such as abstract reviews. Committees with high work burden, like organizing a conference, are not usually a good place to start, especially early in your career when you have grants to write and papers to publish in your pursuit of tenure.

One type of committee that can offer particular learning opportunities is serving on a committee that gives awards within the society. In this type of committee, you have the chance to understand what is considered true excellence in your field. Another committee to consider is abstract reviewing, as it will help you hone your abstract skills by serving as a reviewer. If you like the committee you join, you can grow your presence and your role over time, which we will address in Chap. 9. If you try it and do not find the work interesting or rewarding, look around for a different area of involvement.

Many societies now have committees and affinity groups that focus on specific groups, such as junior members, women, BIPOC individuals, and LGBTQI+ people within the field. This approach is an important way for professional societies to include and recognize diverse members and promote the excellence that comes from diversity in science. Look for this in your professional society, and if it interests you, join!

Contribute: Another benefit of membership in professional societies is the opportunity to engage in positive change or advocacy within your field. The central position of professional societies can bring leverage to design and promote evidence-driven change, including through publications, policy statements, committees, and awards. Keep an eye out for these opportunities, such as contributing to the writing or review of a policy statement, or contributing to advocacy efforts offline or via social media.

What if I Have More than One Professional Society?

It is not unusual for an academic clinical researcher to have more than one membership to large professional organizations. If this makes sense in the scope of your work, and you can afford the dues, these memberships may provide different things at different times in your career. It may be helpful to you to prioritize these societies to determine how much you can give to each, so that you do not end up overstretched. For example, you would want to focus your committee involvement in your main "professional home" and attend that meeting yearly, while your secondary organization you may attend every other year and choose a committee with minimal work. These are useful conversations to have with your colleagues or mentors to learn and consider different strategies.

Meaningful Moments
The Endocrine Society has had a huge impact on my career! By getting involved in the Endocrine Society, I made many new contacts and had opportunities to serve on committees and in leadership committees. These activities were not only helpful for academic promotions at my institution, but also exposed me to models of leadership and leadership styles that I could apply to my leadership roles at my own institution. These activities were also very helpful for networking on a national level, and made the national meetings much more meaningful and integral to my development. Most of all, I have made many important friendships through these activities!

In addition to the Endocrine Society, I have been very active in Women in Endocrinology—this group again provided both formal and informal leadership training, networking opportunities, and wonderful friendships as well as role models. I can honestly say that I would not be where I am today without the Endocrine Society and Women in Endocrinology.

—Ursula Kaiser, MD.

Attending Scientific Conferences

When trying to explain the appeal of the yearly research conference to a non-academic colleague, that colleague commented that it sounded like a combination of a science fair and a nerd prom. Not a bad characterization! Yes, you get to show off your own project and learn from others' projects. Yes, you get to dress up and parade about a bit. Yes, it can be social, including after-parties and the chance to stay up late. Yes, comfortable shoes are important as you will be on your feet a lot. But…. no corsages, dance music or dates are needed (Fig. 5.2).

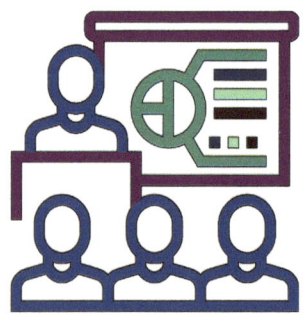

FIGURE 5.2 Attend a scientific conference

Conferences can be rejuvenating. They can be inspirational and energizing opportunities to connect to the greater scientific community. You can step back from the daily management of your own projects and contemplate the bigger picture of where your science is heading. It has been said that a good conference has the capacity to bring a scientist, no matter what career stage, out of a slump.

Strategies to Get the Most Out of Your Yearly Conference

Before You Go

One obvious way that conferences can provide you a chance for rejuvenation is by leaving your everyday routine, traveling to a conference, and immersing yourself in that event. This makes a conference like a mini-sabbatical. Thus, before you go, do your best to "clear your plate." You do not want to show up to the conference with so much work to do that you feel like you cannot leave your hotel room. Clean up your inbox and set your out-of-office messages. Make a list of what you need to get done emergently, and get it done before you go. If you are a clinician, get your charts up to date, and let your clinical staff know who to contact while you are away. Anticipate any deadlines that will happen during or just after the conference, and get this stuff done!

Have your Elevator Speech

You will likely meet a lot of new colleagues and peers at a conference, and mastering the art of your introduction is a key part of these communications. A common introductory statement is "**tell me about your work**." When people ask that, they do not want a dissertation, they want a brief summary. Make sure you can describe your work and area of research within about 2 min. This is your "elevator speech." (Fig. 5.3).

Remember, the elevator speech usually includes a brief statement of your expertise/area of study and your research focus. Some people like to include a statement of a project they are currently working on. Your mission statement from Chap. 2 helps you craft this introductory speech, and you developed this for your informational meetings with new colleagues at your home institution in Chap. 3. A few examples are below (Fig. 5.4):

FIGURE 5.3 Tell me about your work

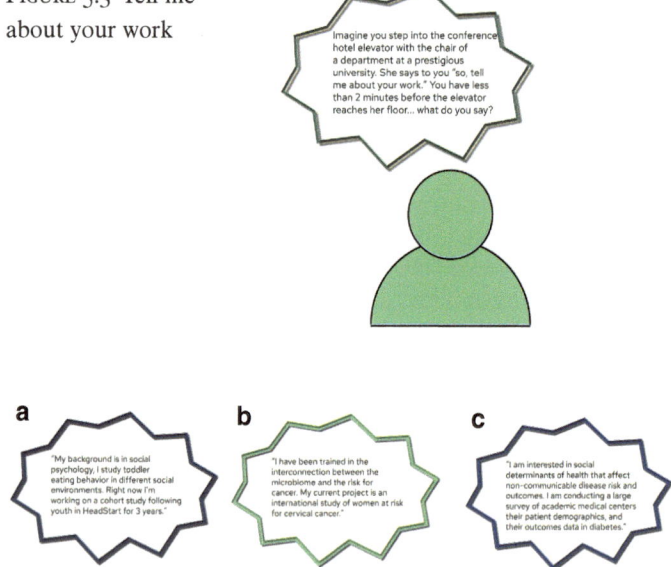

FIGURE 5.4 (**a**, **b**, **c**) Example "elevator speeches" to have at the ready

Know Your Must-Go Sessions

It is a good idea to look over the conference agenda and identify any sessions you feel you must attend well in advance. This may include a presentation by a colleague or mentor, or a key learning session addressing a topic you need to know. Get those on your calendar first.

Stay Centered in Yourself and Your Values

OK, we'll be honest. A conference setting can provide the opportunity for drama. You get a few hundred smart, ambitious type A personalities wanting to show off their stuff, and there can be the opportunity for competition, undercutting, or upstaging. Some ways to avoid that are to reflect on your own values that you bring to the conference, remembering that you can stay centered. You can also talk with your mentor or peer mentor about any experiences you have that concern you. It can be helpful to debrief or decipher an interaction that felt concerning so that you don't let it bother you and ruin your conference.

Meaningful Moments

At academic conferences, there can be subtle or overt interpersonal dynamics that I haven't always been sure how to navigate. These can include male-female power dynamics, female-female power dynamics, or competition between junior faculty who don't yet feel established in their field. Particularly in non-medicine fields (e.g., psychology, communication studies), where tenure hinges on distinguishing yourself as having developed a certain conceptual model or being prominent in a certain topic, the competition can feel pretty intense. Even with junior faculty physicians at the same level as you, the line between competition and comradeship can be blurry, and this is also hard to navigate. I've found it

helpful to talk with my mentor about these experiences - both before conferences and to debrief after-
wards. She has given gentle advice to avoid being the
over-competitive junior faculty, because this can be
off-putting to others, and she always recommends being
intellectually curious, generous, skeptical (even of your
own ideas), and humble (but not overdo it). I've also
asked her for "inside scoop" or demystification of political processes/unspoken rules in academic circles—finding a mentor who can demystify these types of dynamics
beforehand is incredibly helpful.
—Jenny Radesky, MD

Set up Some Coffee Meetings

If there is a mentor or role model you have wanted to meet,
a national conference is a great place to have a 30-minute
coffee meeting. It is entirely normal and acceptable to reach
out to someone before the conference and express interest or
admiration for a senior colleague's work and ask to meet. You
can leverage the same strategies you used in your informational interviews with potential mentors (see Chap. 2) at
conferences, using phrases such as "I'm interested in hearing
about your work," "Can you tell me a little about your training and how it led to your area of research focus?" or "I'd
love to learn about your research." In turn, be ready to provide a succinct description of your work. If there are any
areas of work or advice or input you would like to seek from
this person, have this ready.

Leave Some Room for Spontaneity

Sometimes you will meet a new colleague and want to connect in person for a meal. Sometimes you will bump into an
old friend and want to grab a drink. Sometimes you will be
struck by a new idea and need some writing time to get it on
paper. Do not overschedule your conference time such that

you feel boxed in without the opportunity for these types of activities.

Pace Yourself

Conferences are busy, hectic, fun and...can be tiring. Take time for what you need to do to rejuvenate yourself. Skipping a session to go for a run. Packing healthy snacks when faced with the dreaded "box lunch." Taking a half day to be a tourist in a new city. Spending an evening with a friend who lives in that town. These are all ways to ensure you come home from the conference rejuvenated rather than exhausted.

You Do Not Have to Do it the Same Way Every Year

Some years you may find lots of sessions to attend, and other years you may focus more on committee work. Some years you may bring your partner or family and dedicate less energy to the conference, and other years you may decide to go solo and stay focused on work. You will grow and change in your years going to conferences, and your strategies and priorities at any given conference can also change and grow.

Lessons from the Lab

OK, we will be honest. One strategy that the two of us, Rachel and Megan, have used at conferences for more than a decade is to room together. About every other year, we are at the same conference. And when we are, we share a hotel room. This practice started when we were junior faculty and wanted to be frugal with our meager conference funds, but we both realized there were other benefits. Debriefing after a long day, checking our experiences with each other, supporting each other before our presentations and yes, deciphering drama from time to time, have all been benefits of the tradition we've built. This arrangement or opportunity may not work for everyone, but we have made it work for us.

Being a Reviewer

Reviewing Manuscripts

Reviewing submitted manuscripts (Fig. 5.5) is a simple way in which you can get involved early in advancing to your scientific field as well as building critical research skills. We all write papers to disseminate our science, and reviewing papers can help you become a better paper writer. It can also expose you to the newest findings that are emerging in your field. Most scientists play a role in reviewing papers during their career, so starting this work early can give you experiences that you can learn from and build upon. Building a strong foundation as a reviewer can also lead to later opportunities (discussed in Chap. 9), such as being on a journal's editorial board.

We would remiss if we did not mention a critical rule of manuscript and grant reviewing. You <u>cannot</u> steal ideas you learned about from reviewing, you <u>cannot</u> "scoop" a project you reviewed, and you <u>cannot</u> talk about or write about submitted or unpublished ideas and data with others. You may only develop additional ideas for your own work. For example, you may learn about a variable you had not thought of in the past that you may want to include in your next analyses, or a new topic to do a literature review on to consider for your next project. But you cannot take a research project someone else did and copy it or share it. You want to rock your own science, not steal someone else's.

How do you know if you are ready to review manuscripts? A first checkpoint is whether you are up to date and in a stable place with your own work. As with grants, you do not

FIGURE 5.5 Manuscript reviewer

want to invest in contributing to other people's work at the expense of your own. A second checkpoint is if you have written a few papers and have a comfort level with writing scientific manuscripts as well as a sense of typical elements of a manuscript from reading the literature in your field. This is another opportunity to talk with your mentors about taking the step of becoming a reviewer.

To learn how to review a paper, there are also resources for help. One great resource is your mentor; you can ask to co-review a paper together as a first step. One way to do this is to review the paper separately and each write up your comments, then meet and discuss together. You do not necessarily have to have your reviews match (that is why journals seek 2–3 reviews for every paper since different reviewers will identify different strengths and weaknesses of the paper), but you want to get a sense of whether your review identified any key issues and was thorough. The scientific literature also includes published papers that describe reviewing papers. Your university or professional society may also have presentations or resources on this.

One good tip to keep in mind is that many junior reviewers feel they need to apply the level of editing to reviewing manuscripts that they would apply to their own. Many junior researchers engage in line by line editing for grammar or phrasing in papers they review. This, dear scientist, is not a good use of your time. It is okay to add comments on this here and there, or highlight areas in which the writing is poor and ask the writer to improve it, but you do not need to function as an unpaid copy editor for every paper you review. Line editing takes time and effort, and you are better off focusing that work on your own papers rather than ones you review. The main role of a reviewer is to address the scientific contribution of the paper to your field. You want to focus on content. Is the research question important? Are the methods appropriate to answer that question? Does the paper cite the relevant literature in your field? Is the discussion appropriate at tying in where the study fits in your scientific field of knowledge? These are your questions as a manuscript reviewer.

To identify opportunities to review for a journal, you can seek out your valued resources in your mentors. You can also let your division chief, research director, or department chair know of your interest; these leaders in your institution may also have connections at journals to help you be tapped for these opportunities. If there is a journal you would really like to review for, you can also contact the managing editor and let them know of your interest. Typically, journal editors will want to know your areas of expertise, in terms of topics or methods, based on your research. Make sure to think about this ahead of time and be able to say, for example, "I study substance use interventions for older adults. I would feel comfortable reviewing papers on substance use behaviors and patterns in adult populations, as well as behavioral interventions." Often professional societies link your subspecialty interests to what you may be asked to review for their associated journals; make sure these topic areas are accurate, and if you can declare your interest in being a reviewer to your society, or as you submit a manuscript yourself, go for it!

In some cases, journals will provide you an opportunity to review and then an Associate Editor will evaluate your review. They will evaluate your review based on the thoughtfulness of your comments, NOT on your ability to generate copious comments or line edit the paper. Doing solid reviews over time, and building a reputation as a strong reviewer, can lead to other opportunities within the journal.

Reviewing Grants

Like manuscripts, as researchers we all write grants; however, the ability to review grants is a critical piece of any researcher's toolbox. At the junior faculty stage, most emphasis is placed on the writing of grants, but seeking out opportunities to review grants can provide the invaluable experience of seeing grants from another perspective—the reviewer. You can take that perspective and see your own grants through that lens, making you a better grant writer. Further, reviewing other grants related to your work can help you see trends in methods or topic areas that are considered important right now by your peers and funding agencies. Thus, these activities allow you early contributions to the larger field of your science, and a leg up on your own science.

How do you know if you are ready to review grants? Again, a first checkpoint is whether you are up to date and in a stable place with your own work. You do not want to review grants at the expense of getting your own grants and papers done. A second checkpoint is whether you have a foundation of methods and topic areas in your field that you are ready to review other people's methods and topic areas. Have conversations with your mentor about this. If you feel you are not ready, check with her whether you *are* truly not ready or whether you are merely falling back on imposter syndrome. Your mentor should be able to help with this consideration. (To be honest, no one ever feels totally expert enough to review other people's grants, but the way to develop that expertise is often just by doing!)

To learn about reviewing grants, there are several sources to help you. A first, as always, are your mentors. You may have a mentor who is willing to sit with you and explain the process, or share experiences from her reviews. A second wonderful source is the NIH website. The NIH website has: summaries and score sheets with metrics for their grants; published grants that are exemplary and are annotated throughout noting why they are excellent; videos (you can also find them on YouTube) showing the review process; and even a mock grant review session video. You will want to develop an understanding of the process of review, as well as the strategies used in reviewing the grants you are assigned.

To find grant review opportunities at an early career stage, it can take some work. You may not be known widely in your field, so people may not be seeking you out for these reviews (yet!). Therefore, you may need to do some searching on your own. A few sources of information or potential to help with grant review include:

Your mentors: Talk with your mentors about grant review opportunities because they may know of these within your department, university, or professional society. There may be opportunities to co-review a grant with your mentor to learn the process.

Your university: If there are center, departmental, university, or institution-based grants at your organization, you may want to reach out to the organizers and let them know of your interest in reviewing. These are often smaller grants with less content burden (i.e. 5–10 pages to review compared to 50–100 pages with NIH reviews) and they meet locally, so there is no travel burden.

Reasons to get involved in reviewing grants or papers	Baloney reasons to delay getting involved in reviewing grants or papers
• Your work, including grant and paper submissions, is reasonably up to date • Your mentors agree this is a good idea • You are at a place that you are excited for new challenges • You anticipate writing some grants in the near future and want to get learn new ways to improve your grant writing	• You do not know enough • You are not senior enough • You do not know every statistical or methodological method available • These activities are only for senior faculty who know everything • You need to be an associate professor to do this type of work

Involvement in Your Local Community: Contribute Where You Live and Work

Local community involvement is another area in which scientists often delay engagement. Many cite reasons such as a lack of expertise or not enough time, but usually you do not need to slow developing some type of connection and contribution. Of course, you want to be mindful of reaching your milestones as a scientist and for tenure, but there is no true barrier or magic time in which community involvement is ideal or allowed (Fig. 5.6).

If you do research that has a focus in the local community, you will likely want to get involved early and build relationships. These relationships will directly inform your studies and methods. These relationships will also provide ways to bring your science directly into the community. However, no matter what your area of scientific focus is, there are opportunities for you to contribute in your community in ways that can engage and inspire you, as well as others.

Students

One area of community involvement to consider is contributing to future scientific careers for other young people. Many universities or institutions host programs for undergraduate

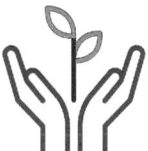

FIGURE 5.6 Community work

students or youth interested in science. These programs may offer opportunities for students or youth to visit the university for a day, or to engage in a summer program providing career exposure to different areas of science. These programs are often seeking scientists to be involved as part of the curriculum. The involvement can vary, but it often includes things like being a speaker on a panel about careers in science, or allowing students to visit your lab. These types of involvement usually take about an hour, which is pretty doable even for a busy junior faculty member.

You can reach out to these types of programs and let them know you are interested and willing to be contacted if opportunities arise. These opportunities can give you new perspective on your role as a scientist, and your capacity to give to a larger community even as a junior faculty. You can be part of engaging and inspiring the next generation of scientists. You can contribute to growing a new cohort of women and gender diverse investigators in science, and advance the excellence that comes from diversity in science.

Community Organizations and Organizers

Another area of consideration for community involvement is in organizations that have shared interests in your area of research. For example, if your research is in LGBTQI+ populations, you may benefit from developing relationships with local organizations that serve these communities. You can contribute by doing a presentation of your work to the organization's staff, or attending a charity event the organization hosts. You may even want to see if you can join the community organization's board. These types of involvements allow you to engage your interest in a shared topic with others from diverse backgrounds. These types of relationships can grow over time in ways that benefit you and the organization.

Another area to consider, depending on your type of research, is to have a community advisory board for your research. Some types of grants, particularly PCORI (Patient-

Centered Outcomes Research Initiative) grants, went so far as to prioritize grant submissions that included a patient advisory board for the project. Typically, you would recruit a group of members from whom you want input on your work, and these may be patients or members of a certain age or demographic group. You arrange meeting times, often quarterly or biyearly. At each meeting, you would provide some updates on your work and ask for feedback. One great way to interact with an advisory board is to present a new study idea and ask for feedback on whether your approach is feasible within the community the advisory board represents. You can then document in your grant or paper that you included this step and input in your processes. Developing an advisory board early on that you can nurture over time can provide you a consistent source of new ideas, reality-checks on your work, and community connections.

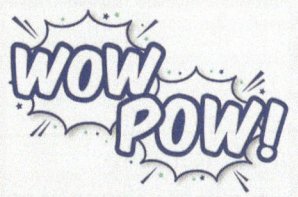

Demi's research focused on health access for elderly people from Native American communities. In order to conduct this research in a scientifically valid way, she knew she needed to learn more about the needs, resources and culture of this community. She first arranged meetings with faculty and staff at her institution to understand best practices in approaching research relationships with specific communities and cultures. Applying what she learned from those meetings, she then approached Native community members, including community leaders and healthcare providers, to request meetings. At those meetings she explained her background and research interests, and asked about the priorities and interests of each person. She emphasized that she hoped for a relationship that was "quid pro quo," in which she could contribute or give back to the community as the community helped her achieve her research goals. It took some time, but over the next 12 months she established a relationship of trust and respect with community members who were willing to help her achieve her research goals. At the community's request, she established an Advisory Board of community members to help guide her research. She offered joint teaching sessions in which she shared information about the research methods she intended to use with the Board, and they shared information about the key cultural practices in the community with her and her research team. She continued her work with the community for many years, honoring their contributions on each poster, presentation and paper, and returning the community to present her findings.

Balancing Multiple Requests

Certain types of research lend themselves more to community involvement than others. Some researchers need to seek out community opportunities that have some connection to their work, others are bombarded with requests consistently. For scientists who have a topic that lends itself to multiple community requests, it will be important to determine an approach on where to put your involvement and time. Talking with your mentor, or even finding a community-oriented mentor to help you decide where to place your time, may be important. It is better to figure out a way to say no, or "not now," if you have too many requests pending.

Take-Home Points

Your outermost circle of your SEM is often the circle that junior scientists struggle with in developing strategies for engagement and meaningful work.

There are several avenues of engagement in the larger community of science to consider early in your career, and foster over time. These include joining professional societies to provide intellectual stimulation and comradery, contributing to the work of science by reviewing grants and papers, and meeting face-to-face with peers and learning from leaders while attending conferences.

We invite you to consider your role in your community, the development of future scientists, collaborating organizations, and your own advisory board.

Homework

- Identify a list of potential professional societies and what they offer (and cost). Review the list with colleagues and mentors to get feedback, begin your memberships with critical professional societies you have selected.
- Develop ideas for committees to join within your professional society, and at your next professional society meeting, attend a committee meeting.
- Investigate opportunities to review grants and manuscripts, identify resources to learn about these skills, create a timeline for seeking these opportunities in the next 2 years.
- Use your research skills to identify opportunities in your community for involvement, reach out to a new organization and see if there is alignment in what you can offer them and what they can teach you.
- If a colleague recommends an organization that aligns with your work, follow up on this by looking into it.
- Consider whether and when an advisory board may bolster your work.

Chapter 6
Your Promotion

This chapter focuses on the requirements for promotion in an academic institution when you are a researcher. We will discuss the process of promotion, and the ways in which you can put your best face forward. An academic research career is long and multifaceted; to that end, it is important to understand what is ultimately of value to your institution and how to match your interests to the requirements and expectations of your job. While you have many roles and goals at your institution, most institutions require you to get promoted, so this is a critical part of your job.

What Is Tenure?

Universities and research institutions typically have different academic tracks for their faculty members. There are often tenure and non-tenure tracks or positions, and it is important that you understand the differences at your institution. Tenure is a term to refer to a long-term faculty position that has no required end date. A non-tenure track position is one that is not guaranteed. That means that you do not always have a guaranteed job in the future. Many universities handle non-tenure positions differently. They also use different

M. A. Moreno, R. Katzenellenbogen, *Women Rock Science*, https://doi.org/10.1007/978-3-031-48418-6_6

names for these positions. Lecturer. Acting. Clinical. Research. Know the terminology.

For those *non-tenure positions*, many institutions require that you agree to a contract on a yearly or every 3 year basis, and included in that is the requirement that you are doing a good job in your non-tenure-track position in order to remain a faculty member. Some require that you agree to a contract on a yearly basis, but they are multiyear contracts, so your annual agreement just rolls you one year ahead. Some designate that you can be in a non-tenure track position for only a set number of years. After that time period, you need to either take a position on the tenure track or you need to find a job elsewhere. You need to do your due diligence to be sure you know what you are agreeing to when you join your university or institution as a faculty member.

For faculty positions that are on a *tenure track*, by definition you are guaranteed a job after achieving tenure, but there can be caveats. Some institutions state that you have tenure, but you may not be guaranteed a full salary in the future despite having a guaranteed job. Some state that you have tenure, but you may have to shift responsibilities, for example, taking time away from research to do additional clinical time if you do not have grant support for a period of time. Again, do your due diligence.

Faculty members on a tenure-track follow advancement, or promotion, from Assistant to Associate to Full professor. The timeline for these advancements can differ at different institutions. Most often the transition from Assistant to Associate Professor is within 6–10 years, and becoming an Associate Professor is where tenure is guaranteed. That timeline can be extended in certain situations, but again this is institution-specific. Having a child can allow you to extend your timeline. Health issues for you, or a loved one, can also allow an extension. If you are making progress, but not quite enough, sometimes a request for a one-year extension is granted to give you some wiggle room. Understand these policies as well.

Many universities require that you go through promotion from Assistant to Associate Professor, but not all universities or all tracks require this. Likewise, many universities require that you go through promotion to Full Professor, but not all. Most importantly, if your university requires that you be promoted, and you do not achieve promotion, you must leave. That is called "up or out." You get one year to find another job after that, and then you are no longer a faculty member at that university. Boom…

Lessons from the Lab
When I (Megan) started as a junior faculty at a large state university, I found the word "tenure" to be confusing and terrifying. I decided to face my fear head-on and made an appointment at the university promotion office within 6 months of starting my job. I met with administrators of the promotion process, who patiently explained the process to me and allowed me to review several binders of previous promotion packets. Once I had seen these and met the people involved at the highest level on campus, it did not seem as scary. Viewing the example promotion packets was incredibly helpful to visualize how I would develop my own systems to keep all that information organized over the next few years.

Know the Tracks and the Lingo

At many universities, tenure track is called just that—tenure track. Other names, or subcategories, for this tenure track include *Clinician Scientist*, *Physician-Scientist*, or *Faculty Scientist*. This track is for people who spend the majority of their time leading independent research projects and the remainder of their time on other academic work, including clinical care, teaching, or administration.

At many universities, there is a second academic track that requires promotion but is not a tenure track. This track is often for physicians who do academic work, but not typically as a majority of their time nor as a principal investigator, or PI. These physicians may focus their academic work on being a clinical research site lead, participating in collaborative projects, working in medical education or administration, or directing quality improvement projects. This type of track carries different names, including *Clinician Educator* or *Clinical Health Sciences* track. These positions typically are on a designated promotion path with specific expectations for productivity to achieve promotion from Assistant to Associate and from Associate to Full Professor. However, these positions may not typically have as high a bar to be promoted as tenure track and also do not confer true tenure. This track can vary substantially by institution, looking very similar to the tenure track at some institutions with substantial protected time and resources for faculty, and looking very different at other institutions with expectations centered on clinical revenue and research time only if it is bought out by grants.

The most clinically focused one. This is typically a non-academic track found at academic medical institutions and is often called the *clinical* track. This is most frequently a non-tenure track position, and it typically does not include any expectations for academic work or research. One university we know calls this track the "*Clinician Clinician*" track (in case there was any doubt to the focus of this track, they say it twice).

A final type of *non-tenure positions* are positions that *do not place you on a specific track toward promotion*. These positions may be called "*acting*" as in "acting assistant professor." Some institutions call these "instructor" positions, as in "clinical instructor." These positions are often a first step toward a faculty position. There are many reasons that an institution offers you this type of position, but since it is a lower-cost and lower-commitment position, it is worth asking questions about why it is being offered to you. Sometimes a university wants to retain you after your training is completed and create a path for you toward becoming faculty, but it cannot offer a full faculty position at the time you are ready for one. Reasons for this may include budget issues or a leadership transition that impedes hiring a full faculty. For example, an interim leader (interim chair or interim division chief) may not have capacity to hire into a tenure-track faculty position. A few things to be clear about if you are offered this type of position include: (a) how long is it anticipated you will be in this position, (b) what are the criteria you need to meet to be offered a faculty position, and (c) what expectations and opportunities you will have for support, including grant support, while you are in this position.

A key piece of information to know is *time limits around when you can switch tracks*. Sometimes faculty are brought in on tenure track and realize it is not the right fit and want to switch to the clinician educator track. There are usually very strict time limits around how long a faculty has to switch tracks and still be promoted, often around 3 years is the limit. Conversely, sometimes faculty are brought in on a clinician educator or non-tenure track position and realize they are better suited to the tenure track. Sometimes a track switch is an important consideration after the first year or two, and you do not want to miss the deadline.

At some universities, a further decision must be made—which promotion committee you want to review your work. At some universities there are separate committees such as biological sciences, social sciences, and humanities. Quite often the clinical and academic work will be submitted for review by the biological sciences committee, but if your work falls on the line between committees, be sure to investigate each committee's priorities before committing to one. Trust but verify.

Create a Mentorship Committee for your Promotion

Many universities require faculty to put together a mentorship committee to support them toward promotion. Even if your university does not require it, it is highly recommended, and we discuss this in Chaps. 2 and 4. The committee is usually made up of 3–5 people with whom you meet to review your progress to date toward promotion and to get their collective feedback. Typically, the committee should be made up of people above you in rank, so if you are an Assistant Professor, these members should be Associate or Full Professor. Some universities choose your committee for you, and some allow you to choose. Selecting your committee can be a challenge, so here are a few helpful hints:

1. Talk to your mentors, other faculty in your division, your division chief, and other people whose judgment you trust to get ideas for who could be on your committee.
2. Consider having at least one member of your committee from outside your division or research center. This will broaden the perspectives of those who are reviewing your work, which is helpful in preparation for the promotion process in which not everyone on that committee will be from your home turf.
3. Try to pick a mix of people more senior to you at various levels (early Associate Professors, later Associate Professors, early Full Professors, senior Full Professors) to represent people who are closer to a recent promotion as well as more advanced in their careers.

Meaningful Moments
The lack of a mentoring committee likely contributed to one of my most painful failures. Despite having grants and publications, I was not promoted in the Basic Sciences Division, which meant I had a year to find another job. However, I didn't have to go far; I was part of a Program Project with people in the Public Health Sciences Division who were outraged at the decision, so a new Program was created and finally a new Division, Human Biology. What seemed awful at the time has turned out to be liberating. I enjoy the more interdisciplinary, translational research that is valued by HB,

rather than only focusing on mechanism. If there is a lesson to be learnt, it is to be resilient. You will definitely have things that don't go your way—a grant not funded, a paper not accepted, a position you want going to someone else—but get over it and move on.
    —Denise Galloway, PhD

Set up your meetings with your committee for regular intervals, at least every 6 months, and contact your committee members to set up the actual meeting about 2 months in advance. Scheduling for a group is always a challenge, so give plenty of lead time to find a date and time that works.

Before the meeting, send out your materials for review (updated CV, annual review form if you have one) a week in advance. Think about whether you have specific questions or concerns to bring to your group.

During the meeting, you will walk through your progress since the last meeting and highlight any areas of significant accomplishment, challenge, or areas you have questions. You will be asked to describe your goals for the short-term (6 months to a year) and longer term (~3 years). You can do this via a slide show (if a virtual meeting), or a review of a document you send out ahead of time. However you want to share this information, be organized and prepared for the meeting. Be sure to take notes during the meeting (or identify a note taker) so you will have a record of what was advised.

How Do you Get Promoted?

Universities advance you up the academic ladder rungs by reviewing the work you have been doing and also by asking others to objectively evaluate your career achievements. To that end, you need to document your productivity in all facets of your job, demonstrating a consistent building of successes that assure you are not only accomplished now, but you will continue to be so in the future. They want to you know you are rocking your science now and will keep it up!

Documentation

To have your best foot forward, you need documentation. Some of that burden is placed squarely on your shoulders, and some is placed on your mentors, bosses, and colleagues. You should save every teaching evaluation, every invited lecture date, title, and location, every mentee's name and degree or project achieved, every review by your mentors or oversight committee, every paper, abstract, and committee membership, and every kudo from a patient or employee. Did we say every enough? EVERY.

> One of the mistakes I have made in my career is the lack of preparation for moving between academic institutions. When I started as a junior faculty member, I was very naive about the types of different tracks in academic medicine institutions, so I focused on the requirements at the institution I started in and the track I started on. Unfortunately, my institutional requirements did not necessitate me to save or catalog much of my work (teaching materials I developed or teaching evaluations I received, learners I had mentored) and after 5 years when I was moving institutions I could not effectively or efficiently recreate this data set. This resulted in the need for additional time for promotion at my new institution and on my new track. Take home message: None of us have a crystal ball about what our futures will look like, though something you have done may not seem relevant here or now, it may be later- so save and catalog it!
> —Shobhina G. Chheda MD MPH FACP

Annual Reviews

You should have *annual formal reviews* with your immediate bosses, be it division chiefs or center directors. These reviews are separate and distinct from your semiannual meetings with your mentorship committee. Your mentorship committee has a role to support and nurture your career, and you meet to create guardrails and smooth roads to assure to make it to your goal of promotion. Your annual reviews with your immediate bosses function as true evaluations of your track record and your chances of future success. The annual review addresses both your everyday expected duties and your scholarly activity.

Before these annual review meetings, it is your job to compile your achievements, and even your failed attempts, over the past year to be able to review how much effort you have been putting into your job and how well it has been going. This allows for a frank conversation about your work and a critical review of your likelihood of reaching the milestones required for promotion. These meetings then should be capped with a summary letter by your division or center director heads as well as your department chairs noting your strengths and next steps. Again, this forms a track record for your larger university to review when its promotion committee reviews your promotion package or portfolio. These annual meetings and letters help you fine tune your progress, and they will form the structure of your promotion portfolio. Documentation is key.

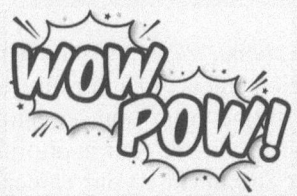

Enid was thrilled as a junior faculty to be asked to be a Medical Director for her community-based clinic focused on refugee health. She invested in meetings with staff, building an Advisory Board of community stakeholders, and setting up curricula for trainees to rotate through the clinic for learning. Her promotion committee included a couple of newly promoted Associate Professors and her Division Chief. Her first few annual review meetings were positive and supportive or her role and her early leadership opportunity where she was clearly investing her time. Enid had her departmental mid-point promotion review after being an Assistant Professor for 3 years. She was surprised when she received feedback that she was considered "at risk" for promotion. She learned that she did not have substantial academic products, such as poster presentations or papers. She realized that to be promoted, she needed to make some changes in how she was working. She sought out a mentor to advise her on how to achieve academic products from her Medical Director job, and soon embarked on several QI projects to assess the systems she was putting in place at the clinic. She added a new member to her promotion committee, an experienced Professor whom she heard had been an asset to other junior faculty's promotion committees. With these changes, she began to build a strong promotion package and get yearly feedback to keep her on track.

While it can be really rewarding to have annual review meetings with committee members who sing your praises, make sure you have at least one committee member who really knows the promotion process for your path, and who will be direct about what areas of your CV need work to achieve promotion. If everyone on your committee is a "people pleaser" or a cheerleader mentor, you could miss out on early identification of gaps in your promotion packet.

Funding

To achieve promotion, documentation is not enough. It is not just paperwork. It is what is IN the paperwork. A scientist in academics needs to demonstrate that she is leading an independent research program. It is important that you are being mentored and supported by your colleagues, bosses, and environment. However, but you must also stand on your own as a faculty member for promotion. At the time of promotion, you are no longer in a career development position, but your career has "developed." At some institutions, that development is based on your bibliography or your funding portfolio. If you have a publication record as a senior author, that demonstrates that you have led a team through a research project. If you have a NIH R series grant where you are the principal investigator or co-principal investigator, then NIH and its study section see you as ready to lead future projects with your research team. These metrics are really important.

Universities and institutions are cognizant of the challenges of federal and foundation funding. Although promotion committees are not necessarily lenient, they are understanding. So, if you are not yet independently funded, but you have tried and been scored well enough that in years past you would have been, reviewers take that into account. Again, know your university's policies and track record.

External Reviews

To achieve promotion, your self-assessment and direct boss's reviews are not enough. You also need to be viewed by colleagues in your field as worthy of promotion. That means you need to get many letters of support, sometimes ten or more, included in your promotion package. Letters will be from colleagues more senior than you, both at your home institution and not, with whom you have and have not collaborated. Some letter-writers may be nominated by you (with advice from your mentors and promotion committee), other letter-writers may be selected without your input. Institutions have specific rules about whether or not you can contact reviewers before the official request, so do not reach out until you have checked these rules.

One thing is common across your letters. They must speak to your achievements and their enthusiasm for your career and future success. You want praise. Respect. Wishing you worked at their university instead of yours because you are JUST.THAT.GOOD.

Mid-Term Review

Some universities have a mandatory mid-assistant professor review to assure you are on-track for the second half of your assistant professorship to be promoted to associate professor. In our opinion, this is a wonderful checkpoint. If your university has a promotion timeline of 6 years from assistant to associate professor, that means you are reviewed at the year three. But it typically takes promotion committees 12–18 months to review your packet or portfolio, comment on it, and have the university extend your assistant professorship for the second 3 years. That means you are being reviewed 18 months into your tenure track position. So, although 6 years may feel like a long time to build your portfolio, 18 months will not.

If concerns are raised during your mid-term review, do not despair, and yet do not dismiss. Some common issues at the mid-term review are not demonstrating enough focus in your work, or not having enough publications or presentations.

Ask tough questions of your committee. Are you not doing enough? Not doing the right things? Doing too much? Take the feedback seriously. You still have time to course-correct at this point. It may be time to evaluate your projects, your mentors, your team, or even your track.

Based on that same lead time, your final evaluation for promotion at year six will be due between year four or five. Again, be aware of the timelines you are expected to achieve, and use your time management skills and academic developments plans from Chap. 2 to meet the milestones you have in place.

The Promotion Portfolio

What do you need in a portfolio? A portfolio is much more than your CV or NIH biosketch. Academics, and academic medicine, includes work in many different aspects of research, education, and clinical care. You need to document your productivity in all of these realms and your successes within those realms.

Some institutions will ask you to designate a major area of your work for the committee to focus on. Sometimes this is called your "area of excellence" or major area of work. For most tenure-track researchers, it is expected that this area will be research. At some institutions you will be asked to designate a secondary area of work, sometimes called your "area of significant accomplishment" or similar lingo. For tenure track, some institutions require this to be in teaching/education, other institutions will allow it to be clinical work, service, or public health. A newer path at some institutions is an "integrated" path in which you can demonstrate that your work contributes across more than one area: research, teaching, and clinical. An example may be a global health researcher who focuses on malaria and focuses her clinical global health work in treating malaria, does research on malaria treatments, and focuses teaching on this topic as well. Know what your options are and when you have to make a determination of your area(s) of focus.

Typically, portfolios are broken into sections that represent these areas of focus. These include (Fig. 6.1):

Promotion Portfolio

Research
- (a) Grant funding
  - (i) Completed, active, pending and future
  - (ii) Direct annual funds
  - (iii) Your role
  - (iv) The main goals

b) Publications
- (i) Peer-reviewed journal articles
- (ii) First author, co-author, and senior authorship

Not hypothesis driven:
- (iii) Review articles
- (iv) Commentaries
- (v) Book chapters

Teaching
- (a) Classes you tought and your evaluations
- (b) Courses you ran and your evaluations
- (c) Courses you developed and your evaluations
- (d) Lectures you gave and your evaluations
- (e) Teaching on the wards and your evaluations

Clinical care
- (a) Board certification
- (b) Licensure
- (c) Time on the hospital wards or in the outpatient clinic
- (d) Clinical evaluations by colleagues, team members, and patients themselves

Administrative work
- (a) Division, center, department, and university committee membership
- (b) Professional society comittee work
- (c) Leadership in a local or national conference
- (d) Clinical programming
- (e) Running a seminar series

Ethos
For many of these sections, universities not only want documentation, but a summation of your work and a description of your ethos. Your personal mission statement that you made in chapter "You as a Scientist" can
be the seed for these statements. Take the time you need to really reflect on why you do research, see patients, teach others, and aid in the infrastructure of your university and professional societies. They want to know.
And you should be able to explain it, creating a framework for your efforts.

Letters of support
- (a) Internal letters: from mentors and colleagues
- (b) External letters: from mentors and colleagues
- (c) Arms-length reviewers
  - (i) Not mentors or colleagues. These letters often carry a lot of weight as they are viewed as objective assessment of your work from people who have not worked directly with you

FIGURE 6.1 Example elements of a promotion portfolio

Arms-length reviewers: From people in your field that are NOT mentors and colleagues. These letters often carry a lot of weight as they are viewed as objective assessments of your work from people who have not worked directly with you. Usually this means someone who has not been involved directly in any of your recent grants or publications. These may be more distant colleagues whose work relates to yours. You may be asked for suggestions of people in your field who are not your mentors or colleagues. Be sure to follow these rules around who is truly arms-length. If you know someone well, or worked on a project with them, they will often mention that in their letter, and this can disqualify their letter or even delay your promotion.

Newer Areas of Focus in Promotion Portfolios

Many institutions are recognizing more areas of work as part of your promotion portfolio beyond the traditional empirical publications and grand rounds style talks. Newer areas of emphasis can include Diversity, Equity, and Inclusion (DEI) work, either at your institution or in the community. Some institutions recognize advocacy, public health, informatics or community health efforts explicitly as areas that "count" for promotion. For publications, non-traditional venues such as blogs, websites, or organizational reports may be part of your package. Also, presentations to community audiences, or media engagement, have been recognized as promotion-worthy types of presentations by some institutions. Know what your institution does and does not recognize for your portfolio. If your institution is reviewing newer additions or criteria, see if you can be part of this important work.

What Happens after your Promotion Portfolio Is Made?

Remember, each university is different. With that caveat in mind, your promotion portfolio will be reviewed by a promotions committee within your department and determined if you merit advancement to the next level of review. After your department agrees on the strength of your promotion portfolio and votes to advance it, it will be sent to the school's promotions committee and then the university leadership. If your university has multiple promotion committees (as noted in the tracks and lingo section), make sure your portfolio is reviewed and evaluated by your ideal one. Most typically, if your department supports your promotion, your school and university will too. It will be signed off by your dean, provost, and president. Then you are set!

What if you are not promoted? Hopefully you had an idea this might happen based on your annual reviews, your meetings with your mentors, and your department's review of your portfolio. If your university has a mandatory promotion timeline, and you do not achieve promotion, you typically have one year to find another job outside of the university. Use this moment to reflect on jobs and positions that are a better fit for your skillsets. Do you enjoy teaching and disseminating data rather than generating it? Do you like advising or guiding ideas more than creating new ones? Do you enjoy mentoring but in a setting different than your current one? You should consider if academic science is the right field for you, but most important, if it is the right job description for you. Everyone can be successful. However, in order to be successful, you need to be in the right job, career, and institution.

Take-Home Points

Promotion takes years to achieve, so research your home institution's guidelines and rules to be ready from the start.

Use your mentoring committee and annual reviews to gauge your progress toward promotion.

SAVE EVERYTHING.

Homework

- Research your institution's tenure-track guidelines and timelines.
- Create a timeline and roadmap to achieve the milestones required for promotion.
- Keep a running list of potential writers for letters of support for your promotion package.
- And again...Save everything! Develop a system on how you will save this information over time.

Chapter 7
Expanding Your Team

In this chapter, we will focus on when it is time to grow, including developing your role as a mentor, growing your research team, and developing collaborations across research groups. The early activities of developing and organizing your research team were covered in Chap. 3. That included seeking mentors, developing a research team, cultivating relationships with colleagues, and leveraging your early experiences as a mentor to others. All of these groups (your mentors, your team, your colleagues) form the innermost circle of your SEM. Chap. 7 therefore represents the next step up. These activities typically are more common at the mid-career level, after you have achieved the early hurdles of career development programs and grants and have a good grasp of your area of research and skillset. Unfortunately, this is often a time when you have less available resources for guidance and information about these important milestones of expansion. So, stay strong! You still can rock your science when it is not just YOU!

Start with Yourself

In this chapter, we focus on the next stages of your work. Rising as a mentor. Growing your research team. Taking on more and loving it. However, this is also a good time to begin

© The Author(s), under exclusive license to Springer Nature   139
Switzerland AG 2024
M. A. Moreno, R. Katzenellenbogen, *Women Rock Science*,
https://doi.org/10.1007/978-3-031-48418-6_7

some self-reflection. There are two key things to consider. First, revisit your passions in science (Chap. 2). Are they the same? Have they expanded, or have they narrowed to a focus area? Ensure your mission statement is up to date and reflects where you are. That way, you can clearly communicate this to others as you expand your team.

Second, reflect on the values that you identified within yourself in Chap. 2. How do those impact your approach to mentoring? Think specifically about your style of mentoring, and how that needs to bend and flex with each individual who makes up your research team.

Third, as you and your team start to grow, think about any new knowledge or skills you will need. Do you need additional training in mentoring, managing people, time management, balancing projects? As you read this chapter, consider how you want to learn these new skills, and how you will create some time to invest in your learning. That will make your bigger team work much better together, synergizing their energy and focus.

You as a Mentor

Remember what you love in your own mentors? They do not try to transform you into a clone of themselves ☹ , but they do help you get where you want to go ☺ . Thus, your role as a mentor for others is not to transform the potential you see in them into your own vision of the ideal. Instead, you must always keep the best interests of your mentees at the forefront.

This can be a difficult shift in thinking, both in keeping the mentee's interests at the forefront and in seeing yourself as a mentor. A first step is to get over the imposter syndrome. You are ready to be a mentor. You can do this!

How do we know you will be a great mentor? Well, you have had a lot of experience as a mentee. You have been there, maybe even recently or presently. You know what values are important in mentoring, such as integrity, trustworthiness, and empathy. You know that the best mentors are not those who know the most, but those who listen and are invested.

WIFM?

What is in it for you is big (Fig. 7.1). Although being an excellent mentor is an altruistic act, it is not one without benefit. You may gain productivity, as your research mentee begins to write papers and present work with your name as senior author reflecting your input and investment in that project. You may generate new ideas for your own work through interactions with your mentee. You may get a feeling of coming "full circle" as a scientist, while once you were the trainee now you can train. This is not déjà vu, but seeing the world from a new and different perspective.

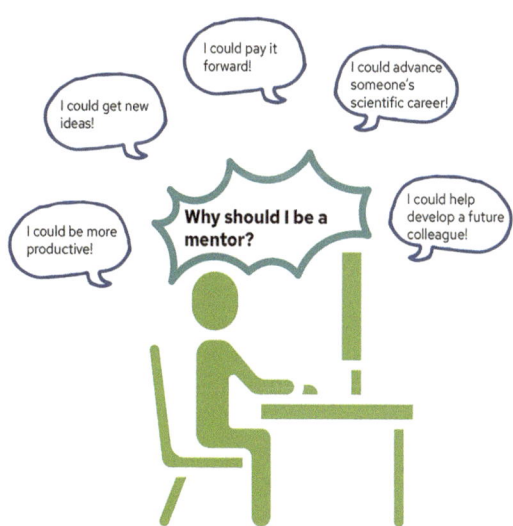

FIGURE 7.1 Why be a mentor?

Lessons from the Lab
Rachel here with an anecdote. I have been lucky to have many good mentors in the hospital and in the lab, but each had specific qualities that I knew I wanted to emulate when I became a mentor myself. I got to practice that early on when I was working as a team member on the hospital wards, and then when I worked at the bench as a fellow. I learned to focus on fostering creativity, staying on task and on time, and letting out the reins when a mentee was gaining skills and confidence. It is very rewarding to see someone become an independent scientific thinker and know that I helped develop that.

Finally remember, you will mentor many different types of people throughout your research career: undergraduates, graduate students, postdocs, and clinical fellows; as well as technicians, research associates, and staff scientists. All of these people, whether working with you for credit or a paycheck, need to be mentored. That approach will foster the very best from them.

When a Potential Mentee Approaches You

Chapter 3 provided an outline of how you can approach potential mentors via background research and initial communication leading into an informational interview. In this chapter, you can consider your role as mentor in that process. The table is turned. When a potential mentee approaches you, be transparent about your availability and interests. If you develop a mentoring relationship with a new mentee, start off on the right foot by establishing your expectations for communication, meeting frequency, agenda, and review time for key documents.

In Chap. 3, we described placing the organization and structure of the relationship squarely on the shoulders of the mentee. Mentees should be in charge of scheduling meetings and setting the agenda. It may be helpful to make your expectations about this clear during an early or initial meeting. In your role as a mentor, you want to foster their independence in this way. This is a skillset that is built only through the absence of something. Your mentees must learn to self-manage their time and their work. You as a mentor will foster that by creating the space to do so. If a mentee seems to be leaning on you to do the structural work (time management, meeting scheduling, etc.) in the relationship, it is time to talk about your expectations for each other. [Nudge nudge wink wink: Perhaps you can refer the mentee to Chap. 3 of this book to ensure your expectations are clear and aligned.]

When Your Mentees Bring You an Idea

When your mentees bring you a terrible idea. First, thank them for bringing this up, and then be honest. Focus on the idea, not on them as scientists. Let them know you are concerned about this idea and give specifics on why. Imagine yourself as a grant reviewer tasked with providing specific feedback on items such as significance, innovation, and approach. Use that structure as a guide for your feedback, based on your mentees' known goals. You can add some positive feedback about them as scientists and your confidence in their ability to rock their science, even if it is not on this particular project.

When your mentees bring you an idea that you are not really sure is good or bad. Let them know you have concerns about the proposed idea (and what they are), and consider suggesting an alternative review from someone with expertise in the topic or methods. Think of this as a second opinion and an opportunity for your mentees to learn skills in seeking consultation and potentially a new additional mentor.

When your mentees bring you an idea that is good or simply great. Recognize it as such, call it out as a fantastic idea. Then allow them to OWN IT and provide them support.

Actions of Effective Mentors

- Provide career guidance. Even if your career is young, you can share your experiences. You can share advice/guidance you were given and how you have or have not used it.
- Be a sounding board. Utilize motivational interviewing techniques more than directed recommendations. Do not try to solve their issues; instead, give them the confidence that they themselves can.
- Help navigate the institution, provide networking, and collect resources. Let them know what is coming in the near future and how you are planning for later.
- Consider sharing data as this provides a low-risk way for mentees to get a research product (as will you).
- When you do not know something as a mentor, that is ok. Studies have shown that good mentors know what their limits are and help their mentees to broaden their network in seeking answers and resources. Remember from Chap. 3, a good mentor is a guide, not a director.

Expanding Your Work Group

Diversity in career stage is a salient driver for my research. My teams usually include graduate students, postdoctoral fellows, undergraduates, medical students, medical residents, and medical fellows. It is important for me to take note of their different career stages because career stage signifies the background knowledge they bring to the team. Their current job title and related career aspirations are also significant because they help me to know whether to assign a team member a short-term or long-term project, and what types of projects to involve them in e.g. clinical or basic science or a combination of both. It will also help me to gauge how much independence I can expect to give them in conducting the research and analyzing and summarizing the results. I also believe it is important to realize that some members of my team need to focus on the "trees" e.g. undergraduates and early-stage graduate students, while others should focus on the "forest" e.g. postdoctoral fellows. Gaining the ability to see both the "forest" and the "trees" is an essential skill that requires time to grow and practice to master.

—Beth Meyerand, PhD

When it Is Time

There are many reasons to expand your research team, the first is the most obvious: you have additional projects, and you need additional staff. Another possible scenario is that you have a great staff, some increased work, and you think your staff would benefit from opportunities to teach, mentor, and enhance their skills. Just as we learn from teaching others, so does your team, so you may be able to elevate their skills by presenting them with additional teaching opportunities through interns or students that they train and mentor. Another scenario is if you would like to diversify your team in terms of skillsets, such as bringing on a staff member who can focus on disseminating your work or someone else with a new set of research skills.

Congratulations, Now You Are a Manager

Once you have expanded your team to a larger number of people, you will really need to think through how you want to manage your team. This is a good time to review the basics of running a team from Chap. 3. Maybe watch a few old episodes of the show "The Office" to ponder Michael Scott and see what bad management looks like (this may motivate you to invest in better skills). Revisit some resources; the One Minute Manager series is a popular line of books that are very short and digestible. Some universities' Business Schools have seminars or workshops on the topic of management. There are even podcasts on building early management skills. We have included some additional resources at the end of the book on management. Whatever your preferred learning style, it is time to ensure you have the skillset to grow and manage your team across a growing number of projects.

Meaningful Moments
Speak with each member, listen to the team. I only hire with input from all laboratory members. They are rarely wrong, in contrast to me. If someone does not function as a team player and is disruptive, do not wait to part ways.
   —Cary Moody, PhD

Ways to Expand Your Work with New Team Members

Idea development: Consider bringing on a student or staff with expertise in a different area of study. For example, if you study medical education, consider bringing on a graduate student or staff with a general education background. If you are studying cellular biology, consider bringing on a student or staff with a background in bioengineering. This cross-fertilization from a neighboring field can bring in new ideas, methods, or theories for your team.

Methods: If you anticipate that you will be using a new method in which you are still getting trained, consider bringing on a staff or student to help bolster your expertise. For example, bringing on a staff or student with specific statistical expertise could mean you will get much more exposure and access to someone who knows that method, compared to infrequent consultations with a statistician. Bringing on a student or staff with specific expertise in biochemistry could help you develop experiments that stretch beyond cellular biology or model system studies.

Dissemination: If your work has opportunities for dissemination, especially non-conventional dissemination such as creating a handout for a patient group or writing a blog, consider a staff or student with background in journalism or communication. There are many opportunities for dissemination through new channels such as social media, blogs, and community content that can increase the reach of your work. While, of course, publication in peer-reviewed journals is still the coin of the realm, having help with this non-scientific-ese type of writing can present new ways to broaden the impact of your work. Further, these skills can also translate into making more creative posters or slides, and honing your elevator speech for future collaborators.

Diversity and Equity

As you consider taking on your own mentees and expanding your own team, it is a good time to reflect on diversity and equity. Diversity in science contributes to better science. Thus, at this transition to expanding your roles and team, it is an opportune time to reflect on your commitment to diversity and equity. There are several ways in which you can enhance your capacity to attract diverse mentees or team members.

Reaching out to organizations or diversity officers on your campus can help you learn best practices in recruiting and mentoring diverse students and junior scientists. These meetings can also provide you the opportunity to establish yourself as an advocate for diversity and equity on your campus. Further, you should review any job or internship postings you publicize to ensure the wording directly addresses your commitment to diversity. You may want to consider cultivating a mentor who is knowledgeable in diversity and equity to enhance your own understanding of the benefits of working with diverse mentees and team members and strategies for your and their success.

> I am aware of who is at the table and who is not at the table. I am happy to prioritize building a diverse, inclusive team. It's easy for everyday questions to take us away from working on bigger priorities, and we put in place standard processes to help us stay on track. Metrics and accountability are important too. A recent NEJM article highlighted that leadership bears that responsibility if we do not build a more diverse workforce — this is something for us to work hard on.
> —Ruanne Barnabas MBChB, DPhil

Cultivating New Relationships with Research Groups

At this point in your career, you may have stumbled upon other groups whose work intersects with yours. Maybe you met an investigator at a national conference and learned that she runs her team very similarly to yours. Perhaps you met a faculty member at a department event and realized your work has more in common with hers than it used to. These scenarios present opportunities to engage your group with another for mutual benefit.

Meaningful Moments
Having strong, meaningful partnerships with other researchers and institutions has allowed us to diversify our funding. With increasingly quick grant turnarounds and specific eligibility requirements, other partnering organizations may be in a better position to apply—matching funding to the assets of each partner.
—Stephanie Craig Rushing PhD, MPH

What Do these Collaborations Look Like?

Across-group collaborations can take many forms. For example, two research groups may partner on an initial project that establishes their work styles and areas of interest. If this goes well, the groups may continue to seek out opportunities to work together. In some cases, staff members on each team may develop working relationships, which can foster enhanced productivity for both groups.

How Do I Foster these Collaborations?

In many cases, these opportunities will happen to you, and it is upon you to take them up. Set up meetings and discussions with the other group to explore project ideas and potential areas of intersect. If you have truly never met another group that you thought you would like to work with, it is likely that you are not getting out and representing your work enough at the institution or national level. You are not hearing about them, and they are not hearing about you!

Some easy steps to foster collaboration are to set up a group meeting by phone or in person. Ask the investigator to invite key members of her team, and you do the same. These meetings often flow well with one group presenting key aspects of its work, and then the other group presents its key areas. In many ways, these meetings flow similarly to "informational interviews" described in Chap. 3. However, it is also an opportunity for group interaction and thus group idea generation.

Try to end the meeting with a set of concrete next steps. For example, maybe there is a grant deadline you want to work toward with a collaborative proposal submission. Maybe you have some data you would like to share for an abstract deadline. These structured tasks give you the chance to really try out working together.

WIFM?

Collaborating across groups presents opportunities for you to expand your thinking and your relationships. It offers opportunities for your research team to feel like a team and work in concert with another group. Your work may have an expanded audience and reach if the other group presents and publishes in areas that differ from yours. Team science is the new ideal in the roadmap of medical interventions, and it is the new way to have excellence and innovation at the National Institutes of Health.

Meaningful Moments

I like Team Science because it exposes you to people who think about things in entirely different ways. In the case of HPV (Human Papillomavirus), I was the Team leader (we were awarded a team science award by American Association for Cancer Research in 2011). In

the case of Merkel Cell Polyomavirus, I am a team player and both roles are rewarding. The Golden Rule is a good principle to follow.
— Denise Galloway, PhD

Time Management

With all of these exciting things to take on and do, it may be time to revisit your time management skills. It is often the case that as you get busier, the strategies you used in the past are no longer effective. If you find yourself cramming writing in during evenings at home, or answering emails at 1 a.m., you may need to reexamine your time management.

One idea to approach this is to set up some meetings with others, focusing on the area of time management. Starting with your mentors, set up a meeting to learn on how they organize their days. You can ask whether they would be willing to look together at their calendars for the week and talk through how they structure it. You can ask what system they use to keep track of tasks. You can ask them how they learned these approaches, and any advice for you to explore.

You can also identify people whom you see as being highly organized, even if they are not your mentors. Let them know you are interested in improving your time management and that you see them as someone who sees to be rocking this.

Your goal is to identify some options and try a few new strategies to see what will work for you. No single person's system is likely to solve everything for you. But you can take pieces of several strategies and weave them together for your own approach.

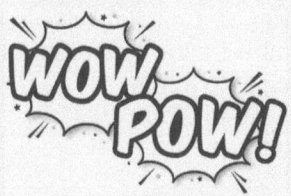

Anisha has been a successful junior faculty, she is an intensive care unit physician and her research focuses on lung volumes in mechanically ventilated patients. Her first few years were marked with success; she achieved a K grant and ran a small team well. She has now transitioned off of her K and has her first R grant. However, she is feeling increasing pressure to find grants to fully fund her research time. She has also taken on the role of ICU fellowship director. Further, her research team now has fellows and graduate students working in it, so it has nearly doubled in size. She finds that she often prioritizes addressing the needs of her team and trainees, and finds herself doing her own work, writing, and analysis late at night. She realizes she needs to revisit her time management structure and how she manages her team.

Time for a Coach?

At this stage of growth and increased demands of you as a manager, leader, and agenda-setter, some investigators can feel like an entirely new set of skills and training is needed. However, the faster pace of your research career at this time point usually means that there is no time to take classes or courses in this area. For some researchers, working with an executive or leadership coach can be a way to refine and hone your management or leadership skills.

Coaches have a variety of backgrounds and skillsets; some have strong experience working with scientists or academicians. Coaches help you identify your learning goals and tailor a mini-curriculum to you. That curriculum may involve assigning readings and then discussing them, creating documents for the coach to review, or even practicing role-playing for tough conversations or scenarios. Remember, coaches are different than mentors. A coach teaches you a new skill or helps you master a skill that you already have. A coach does not direct your work nor formally guide your career.

Thus, working with a coach can provide you tailored learning and skill-building for the next stage of your career. Coaches provide a confidential and safe place to take risks in your learning. The downside is that coaches can be expensive. This is not an altruistic affair. In some cases, faculty choose to invest personal funds in pursuing career coaching. In other cases, faculty may have institutional or seed funds to cover this. Finally, faculty entering a leadership position in their institution (see the next chapter) may have funds to direct for specific leadership training. All of these are important to consider.

If you decide to consider working with a coach, use your research skills. Investigate options in your area and conduct informational interviews with at least three to four coaches. Find out their availability, flexibility, and experience with what you want to learn. Set expectations around meeting frequency and their availability to help you troubleshoot in between meetings by email or a phone call. Your coach takes on a role of trusted advisor, so you want to know all you can before investing in that person. The investment can be a career-changer, so some up-front research is necessary.

Take-Home Points

Your innermost circle of your SEM remains critical to your productivity and success as you move further into your career. Just as in the early part of your career, you need to schedule time to consider your needs, strengths, and opportunities. Invest in cultivating your role as a mentor, the growth of your team members, and a new understanding of yourself as a leader and manager of your team and work. Consider investing in your own growth through learning new skills and potentially working with a coach.

Homework
- Consider your availability for serving as a mentor:
  - Reflect on your research mission and where mentorship fits within it.
  - Create some guidelines around what areas of work you are ready to provide mentorship and how it would fit in your schedule.
- Develop a plan for your research team size and structure with 3-year goals in mind:
  - How will you grow to get to those 3-year goals?
  - If you are interested in drawing students or staff with particular skillsets, set up meetings with colleagues in those departments to encourage them to send students your way.
  - Review your annual development plan as a part of these goals (Chap. 2).
- Create a plan to develop new relationships with other research groups.

Chapter 8
Your Institution: Growing Within

In this chapter, we will explore the idea of growth and leadership positions within an institution. This is growth within your own context, where you are not only leading your own team as a scientist but you are becoming a leader of other leaders. In the Socioecological Model described in Chap. 1, these are the second (and third) circles of context around the individual (ME).

What Is "Growing"?

As you move through the academic hoops as a scientist in the medical field, you will mark milestones in your career. They are noted on your CV. They are documented in your annual reviews. They are displayed on your research group's landing page. These hoops allow you to be promoted from Assistant, to Associate, to Full Professorship within your institution. These promotions are based on achieving expected goals within a set period of time. These achievements are relatively consistent across academic institutions, in that your peers from across the country also pledge that your work would merit promotion at their home institutions (A review from Chapter 6 focused on promotion is provided below in Fig. 8.1).

Some institutions have an "up or out" policy for promotion. That means you must achieve your expected goals for

© The Author(s), under exclusive license to Springer Nature Switzerland AG 2024
M. A. Moreno, R. Katzenellenbogen, *Women Rock Science*,
https://doi.org/10.1007/978-3-031-48418-6_8

Promotion Portfolio

Research

(a) Grant funding
  (i) Completed, active, pending and future
  (ii) Direct annual funds
  (iii) Your role
  (iv) The main goals

b) Publications
  (i) Peer-reviewed journal articles
  (ii) First author, co-author, and senior authorship
Not hypothesis driven:
  (iii) Review articles
  (iv) Commentaries
  (v) Book chapters

Teaching

(a) Classes you tought and your evaluations
(b) Courses you ran and your evaluations
(c) Courses you developed and your evaluations
(d) Lectures you gave and your evaluations
(e) Teaching on the wards and your evaluations

Clinical care

(a) Board certification
(b) Licensure
(c) Time on the hospital wards or in the outpatient clinic
(d) Clinical evaluations by colleagues, team members, and patients themselves

Administrative work

(a) Division, center, department, and university committee membership
(b) Professional society comittee work
(c) Leadership in a local or national conference
(d) Clinical programming
(e) Running a seminar series

Ethos

For many of these sections, universities not only want documentation, but a summation of your work and a description of your ethos. Your personal mission statement that you made in chapter "You as a Scientist" can be the seed for these statements. Take the time you need to really reflect on why you do research, see patients, teach others, and aid in the infrastructure of your university and professional societies. They want to know.
And you should be able to explain it, creating a framework for your efforts.

Letters of support

(a) Internal letters: from mentors and colleagues
(b) External letters: from mentors and colleagues
(c) Arms-length reviewers
  (i) Not mentors or colleagues. These letters often carry a lot of weight as they are viewed as objective assessment of your work from people who have not worked directly with you

FIGURE 8.1 Example elements of a promotion portfolio

promotion within a conscribed period of time. It is mandatory. You are either promoted (UP) or you must leave (OUT). Other institutions have non-mandatory promotions or categories of faculty paths that never require promotion. We discuss these pathways in more detail in Chap. 6, and it is important to understand these policies when you accept a position as an academic scientist.

However, as you move through these academic hoops, you should also pay attention to something else. You may discover new qualities in your work that you really enjoy. These qualities are not topic-based. They are context-based. Do you enjoy mentoring in your research group? Do you enjoy giving seminars to a diverse audience, explaining your science so everyone can understand? Do you like working with teams to develop streamlined approaches to research questions? Do you like talking with colleagues about strategies to develop their own careers? Do you enjoy working with others to increase the rigor of their research and scholarship? (Fig. 8.2).

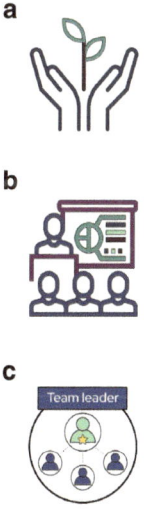

FIGURE 8.2 (**a**, **b**, **c**) Examples of ways to contribute to your institution including community work, presenting at national conferences and leading your research team

You have been trained to do independent research. That keeps you focused on executing on your own research projects. That assures that you can move up the tenure ladder. Achieving these goals, in and of themselves, should be immensely satisfying. However, still it is important to attend to these quality-based revelations about your work too. These revelations can be subtle. With attention though, you can seed a spark in your career, and that spark can grow into a new fire of interests. These interests will grow your leadership beyond the singular, yet fundamental, work of independent research questions.

You (hopefully) enjoy the work you do in your career. A life doing great science is a life well lived! That individual work, and its personal advancement, is always your goal. For a few, the development of others is an additional goal — so much so that they add growing within their institution to advance the careers of others. This may be a goal for you too.

So, you will need to do excellent research and rock your science, but you also will need to pay attention to new skills that you have. These skills may be ones you never knew you had until you take the time to reflect. They may also be interests you never knew you enjoyed. Until you develop your own research, and spend real time in an academic institution, you likely will not have learned how well you could execute and lead team-oriented work.

Below we will discuss some of the different categories of leadership positions that an institution typically has. Some of these may speak to you, while others may not. Reflect on what these positions entail and think, "Would that be me?" Regardless of your own interest in growing within your institution and gaining leadership roles, you need to know what these positions do. If you do not grow into them, others will. You may end up on the search committee that picks the best candidate for the job. And that candidate will become your boss!

Who, me? (Fig. 8.3).

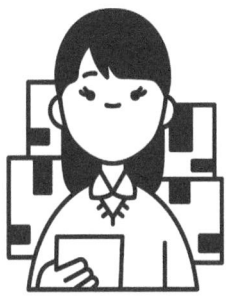

FIGURE 8.3 CEO

Some women and gender diverse scientists struggle with the idea of becoming a leader in their institution, perhaps wrestling with the "I can't do this, I am…" (fill in the blanks: not senior enough, not what they are looking for, too shy, too talkative, too restrained, not restrained enough). This phenomenon is similar to "imposter syndrome," in which people in leadership positions feel like they are an imposter in the role. It is easy for us to write that you should shake off these feelings. There are more men leaders than women, trans, or non-binary leaders in science, and the time is overdue to change that. Do not let this history define your path. But these words are easy to write, and we are all scientists here, so do not take our word for it…collect some data.

Meet with your innermost circle, your mentors and promotion committee. Talk with them about your interest in potential leadership positions and which may be good matches for you. Collect this data, analyze it, and determine your planned intervention.

Meet with those at your institution, those who are in leadership positions you may want to step into in the future. Ask about their paths and input on strategies to prepare for leadership roles. Collect this data, analyze it, and include your findings in your planned intervention.

Meaningful Moments
Being shy does not pay off; I tried it.
— Suzanne Wells, PhD

It is also important to realize that the right position and right timing may not always align. You may identify a leadership position for which you think you are perfectly suited, and then see it be given to someone else. Conversely, you may be nominated for a wonderful position for which you are not sure you are ready. Moving up or along in leadership does not always follow a logical path in the moment. It can feel at times like the old board game Chutes and Ladders. Leaning into your SEM and your skills will help you immensely in these efforts.

Meaningful Moments
I don't think I have ever felt ready for an additional leadership role but fortunately I had learned early in my career that "feeling" ready wasn't a pre-requisite for truly being ready. I do think that the way we trained in medicine in the care of patients was helpful in developing this mindset. I have relied on the trust of the people around me to judge my preparedness and skill. I often tell myself when I apply for a position- "If I don't have the skills or am not the right person for the position, I won't be offered it- and that is ok". I guess the real readiness needs to be about readiness for rejection.
— Shobhina G. Chheda, MD MPH FACP

Types of Leadership Positions Within Your Institution

Department, Division, and Section Chairs

A chairperson of a section, division, or department is a *leader of colleagues within the same field of work*. This work is typically focused on a shared clinical skill or research area. For example, a *department chair* of immunology leads faculty members who are all studying immunology and the immune system. This may include MD, MD PhDs, or PhDs, but they are all members of the same institution, follow the same promotion track, and have the shared goals for their teaching, training, and research. Most department chairs are supported by Vice-Chairs. Vice-Chair positions typically serve "at the pleasure of the chair" and are the chair's own personal leadership cabinet. Vice-Chair roles can include a Vice-Chair of Research, Vice-Chair of Clinical Affairs, and Vice-Chair of Education, to name a few standard ones. Some departments have other Vice-Chairs, such as focusing on Academic Affairs, DEI, or Community Health. These senior leadership positions often arise from dedicated excellence and going beyond one's lab or division work in your contributions. Getting to know your own vice-chairs in your department is a great way to learn about these roles and get exposure to the type of work these roles involve.

A *division head* or *division chief* leads a subset of faculty members who work within one department. They are a group of people who share a narrower focus in their clinical care, teaching, training, or research. Some large divisions, such as general pediatrics or hospitalist medicine, may have an academic division chief and a clinical division chief. Further, sometimes a large division, such as general pediatrics, may have a section within it, such as sports medicine. These groups may have both a division head of the full division and a section head for the smaller group. Within a section or division, there may be a narrowed focus to their work, but there can also be a broader array of member types. For example, an adolescent medicine division head may lead faculty members who all care for and do research about people in the second decade of life. However, because adolescent medicine is very multidisciplinary, the division head may lead MD, MD PhD, and PhDs as well as social workers, nurses, dietitians, clinic managers, case managers, and outreach workers.

As a leader of a section, division, or department you must be interested in the development of others. Your job is to lead all people under you on their best path. You identify skills and help strengthen them. You identify and address gaps in your division or department portfolio by inviting new members. You facilitate transitions for people who will be more productive in different roles or institutions. You coach. You mitigate. You advocate. And you let people go.

In addition to developing others, you develop research, clinical, and educational programs. This development comes from outside members joining your ranks or raising the skills of people already under you. You see what is on the horizon in your field, and you move your section, division, or department forward, becoming leaders nationally. Your work must be visionary, and your style must inspire and support your members to strive toward that vision. Pragmatically, you must also follow the money. Managing budgets that include grants, faculty salaries, clinical programs, and teaching workshops are a big part of executing a vision.

Finally, as a leader, you direct your members in order to train future leaders in your field. You assure your researchers mentor graduate students, postdoctoral fellows, undergraduates, medical students, and residents in cutting-edge work. You also assure that they mentor with the strength and support needed for trainees to become independent themselves. Your work as a leader is more indirect than that of a faculty member leading your own research team. In this leadership role, you mentor the mentors. This is fundamental in any academic institution. It is the cornerstone of science.

Meaningful Moments

I did not have "Division Head" on my 5- or 10-year plan; however, it soon became clear to me that if I wanted to have impact on the pediatric pulmonology community as well as impact on the careers of women and underrepresented minorities in medicine (URiM)—I would need to have a bigger platform. I have been a Division Head now for over 5 years, and it has been incredibly rewarding work. I have the opportunity to mentor junior faculty and provide them with the tools and resources to excel in their chosen path, which I love to do. I also have the opportunity to be a role model to those around me, just by showing up as my authentic self every day. Because of my interest in diversity, equity and inclusion initiatives, I have also taken on additional leadership roles in academic professional societies in order to provide mentorship and new initiatives to support the careers of URiM.

— Terri Laguna, MD

Deans

A dean *leads department chairs within a school* at a university, and a dean also works with assistant and associate deans within the school who can lead students, faculty affairs, curriculum, and research. A dean typically is chosen from a national pool of people who already have led a department. So, you need to have demonstrated leadership skills and significant experience already in place to be considered for a deanship.

The development of faculty is more indirect when you are a dean. You guide your department chairs in their work, but you do less individual, direct mentoring of individual faculty as a dean. Rather, the balance of your work turns to program development, budget management, and the broad oversight of education within your school. Program development and budget management go hand-in-hand; funding for a school comes from student tuition, endowments, state support, clinical revenue, and research dollars. In turn, each of these streams of revenue is tagged for use. If little money comes to a school for research, there are pinch points for program development in research. If a lot of money comes to a school from endowments or gift funds, there may be stipulations on their use. If your school is greatly underwritten by clinical revenues, then growth of clinic space may be critical. As the dean, you create and support the focus of your school, and the departments within it. You work with your university to grow and guide that, with dollars in mind.

As a dean, by overseeing your school's education, you affect people who are just beginning to train in your field. In that sense, you will shape the *future* of your field much more directly than by mentoring junior faculty. You open doors to students just learning about and deciding on their future careers, and you will write or oversee the creation of letters of recommendation for every single one of them! Students will come to you with questions, and they will ask for advice and guidance. They will model their careers on the faculty, trainees, and staff that they see during their school years. As a dean, your school may emphasize diversity, rural health care, research, public health in low-resource settings, or excellent experiential education. The students who graduate from your school will be marked by those experiences and see their future work through that lens. You color that lens.

Associate or Assistant Deans typically have a specific area of focus in their work. One example is an Associate Dean of Faculty Affairs who may focus on areas of professional development or academic advancement for faculty across a medical school. Another example is an Assistant Dean of Students who may focus on issues that arise for medical students. The paths to these types of positions often involve demonstrating leadership and excellence in that topic area of work. For example, an Assistant Dean of Students may have previously served as a department's director of medical students, or vice-chair of education. An Associate Dean of Research may have contributed to leadership on grant reviews, mentoring programs, or multicenter trials. These are positions that are worth exploring through your mentor committee, or meeting with leaders in these positions to understand their path.

Meaningful Moments

What I most enjoy about my work as a leader in academic medicine is being part of driving the mission forward—to alleviate suffering and improve health. I find this deeply meaningful; it's what gets me up every day and fosters my continued joy at work. I once heard it said that academic medicine is a national treasure, and that has always stuck with me. My leadership role is predominantly to support the faculty that make up the heart of the academic medicine workforce: the investigators, clinicians and educators that carry the missions on their shoulders. There are certainly easier careers; a life in academic medicine is demanding, rife with setbacks and frustrations amidst the discovery, impact, rewards, and enjoyment - it requires great resilience and persistence. I appreciate the opportunity to be part of, and to support, such a community of purpose.

—Mary Dankoski, PhD

High-Level University Leadership

University leadership positions vary by campus and can include provosts, chancellors, and associates affiliated with these positions. Universities vary in how they approach these positions, but they can be highly valuable ways to use a management skillset and build on leadership positions.

Meaningful Moments

I felt like being a Vice Provost for Faculty and Staff Affairs was a logical next step for me on my career path. It utilized the skills and experience I gained as a Department Chair and allowed me the opportunity to work on issues that span the entire campus. I found I really enjoy this 30,000-foot view of campus, which is something that even the Deans do not have. I also enjoy helping people reach their career goals, and the Vice Provost role allows me to do that for all the faculty and staff on our campus. It also involves a lot of policy development and review, and those are activities I engaged in and enjoyed when I was Chair of the Executive Committee of our Faculty Senate.

I was fortunate in that I knew the person in the Vice Provost for Faculty and Staff Affairs role when I applied for the job, so I was able to ask him what his day-to-day activities were and what preparation he thought was best for the role. Those conversations gave me confidence that I had the background required for success in the role and that the work would be enjoyable and fulfilling.

—Beth Meyerand, PhD

Research Center Director

As the director of a research center, you wear a different hat than someone who leads a section, division, department, or school. Your mandate and scope are topic-based, not discipline or training-based. Therefore, your work may cross many divisions and departments when you run a center. You develop the portfolio of research ideas and topics within your center, you foster collaborations and cross-disciplinary projects, and you help remove barriers that slow the generation of novel data. Your mandate is to accelerate the development and execution of research, which is a component of a faculty member's career, but rarely it is the full focus of a career. You recruit new members to your center that complement the work and expertise of members already in place. You also help formulate larger program project grants and consortium grants that interconnect researchers and create infrastructure that streamlines science.

Like division and department heads, as a research center director your work will be driven by budgets. Money coming into your center through research dollars will support not only the scientific projects of the principal investigators but the faculty, trainees, research technicians, clinical associates, administrators, and grants managers who touch this work day in and day out. You will mentor the faculty within your center, you help guide their work and the collaborations that are feasible among them, and you grow your programming based on the direction of your cohort of members. Your mentoring will be in complement to that from a faculty's home department, but rarely in place of it. It is exciting to support and accelerate research done by faculty. It is exciting to train future researchers studying within your center's research teams. It is also exciting to identify and work toward collaborative research projects than can only come from the shared partnership of ideas and expertise within your center.

Interdisciplinary Research Team Leader

An interdisciplinary research team leader is different than a research center director. Rather than heading a center focused on a topic and or a scientific discipline, you are the leader of a team that is cross-disciplinary. There are lab-based, patient-based, and population-based researchers that you lead on a collaborative, topic-specific project. You help stimulate the ideas, make the connections, oversee the projects, and assure completion of your goals. Your role as a team leader is both intimate and indirect. You directly oversee the work (and budgets) of investigators on your team and project, but you also dictate the pace and benchmarks for your shared work that is much more administrative. This type of leadership position is the future for health and biomedical research, but it remains a challenge in our current funding climate and training paradigm. Very often this leadership position is termed. You lead a group based on the funding for a project, and once the funding is spent, your group separates. However, strong teams can be maintained to lead serial projects, and that history of excellence in interdisciplinary research is a critical quality to achieving future work. Being adept at leading interdisciplinary research teams is a quality that you should foster!

Administrative Clinical Management

Management of clinical programs is critical for seeing patients who need excellent medical care. You decide what the focus of your clinic is. Do you see patients for weight management? Well care? High blood pressure? Procedures in clinic? Referrals only? Do you have physicians only or mid-level providers too? Do you have multidisciplinary teams in your clinics? Social workers? Nurses? Medical assistants? Phlebotomists? Do you have medical students all day? Two days a week? Are you a training site? Do you have preceptors? How quick is your clinic pace? How do you use electronic medical records? How many research protocols will you allow in your clinic site?

As a director of clinical programs, you define the scope of work expected by your practitioners. In large health organizations, you may be charged with translating and implementing larger system priorities. You identify pinch points for patient flow and for faculty work. You review gaps in clinical care that need to be met in your clinic and help fill that gap. You advocate for space, team members, and adequate reimbursement for the care you all give. And you live and die by your budgets. Like most other leaders, you must balance your spreadsheets to maintain your faculty, trainee, and staff's productivity. This type of leadership position is not typically filled by someone with a strong research focus, unless it dovetails well with your research area. Be careful of taking on a job with such a big clinical focus if your passion lies in research.

Administrative Educational Leadership

Do you love teaching? Does the inspiration of others fuel you? If so, then educational leadership may be a good fit for you. As academicians, you are trained to do independent work well. However, you are given few skills in how to teach or train others—either in didactics or in experiential learning. You may be dynamic in one-on-one mentor–mentee relationships, but standing in front of a lecture hall filled with sleepy graduate students is intimidating. Many people go into academics because they love training people—be it in clinical care or research. However, there are a few who love teaching and the development of excellent curricula and programs that speak to the next generation of leaders. Exceptional educators are fundamental to academic science. No one will want to study epidemiology, biology, or implementation sciences if her class on that topic was boring. As an academic education leader, you can hone your skills in distilling the fundamentals of a subject for new learners. You can delve deeply into a specific topic in intensive seminar-based classes. And you can create a multiyear, structured curriculum to lead a student from being a novice to an expert. Finally, as a researcher, you will develop educational resources that are evidence-based and formed with rigor. Academic institutions are mandated to train and to teach. Leading faculty in best practices for didactic and practicum work is selfless and extremely fulfilling. You will teach the teachers. And you will teach the future teachers too.

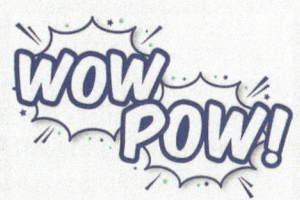

Every year Jules teaches three lectures to the second year medical and graduate students on cancer biology. They get great reviews, and they enjoy returning to the classroom where they get to teach pathophysiology and also discuss current science articles. Jules asks the course director if there are opportunities to lead the course or curriculum for these students. Indeed, the current director is going to take a sabbatical next year, and Jules gets the opportunity to not only teach the course for the entire quarter, but they also are given salary support to restructure the class with more a more dynamic "flipped classroom" approach. They love the work, and the students are also engaged enough that two of them want to rotate with their research group. Jules was asked to share their methodology with to the three other faculty members who teach similar required classes. Now, a class that had notoriously bad reviews for the first time is getting higher marks by its students.

These types of roles may also include leadership over a training program that involves leadership. For example, the National Research Service Award (NRSA) fellowship program provides research training for primary care fellows in pediatrics, internal medicine, and family medicine. Being a fellowship director for a program such as this is an Educational Leadership role, but in a research area. Some residency programs have resident research directors, which is another example of an educational role that focuses on research training, teaching, and mentoring. Finally, an excellent researcher who also enjoys predoctoral and/or postdoctoral training can lead a training grant. These grants typically are funded through national organizations (NIH) and support a specific topic (infectious diseases, oncology) or a specific type of trainee (minority physician-scientist). Some grants fund any person training in research (MD, PhD, MD PhD) and others fund trainees across many disciplines (social work, psychology, medical, nutrition, and nursing). As a program director of a training grant, you oversee didactic training, research projects, faculty mentors, and career development of those funded by the training grant. Your success is based on your trainees' successes. If they become researchers themselves at academic institutions, you have done your job. Congratulations!

Administrative Faculty Development Leadership

What if your skills lie on the soft side? What is "the soft side," anyway? Soft skills are those that are not easily taught in the classroom or at the bench. They are not the WHAT or the WHY but the nuance and subtly of the HOW. How do you learn? How do you teach? How to you mentor? How do you lead? A leader in faculty development focuses on the training and support of faculty members within a department or school. That development lies outside of the faculty's individual research scope, administrative roles, or clinical care. If you lead faculty development, you will develop and execute curriculum on mentoring, health and wellness, mindfulness, diversity, equity, and inclusion, and work–life balance. You may also have a corollary to your work—faculty remediation. That is, oversight of faculty who have acted in error and require directed oversight. That is a challenging role, but the broad development of faculty in an academic setting is exciting and can dramatically expand the support members feel in the growth of their careers. This is reflected in the academic environment of an institution, discussed in Chap. 4.

Other Administrative Leadership

There are other areas of leadership within your institution, and keeping your eyes wide open is one way to identify and explore these areas. Here are a few examples of opportunities that may appeal to academic clinical researchers:

1. Institutional Review Board leadership: Every researcher will interact with the IRB, but some researchers will engage more and seek leadership within this committee.
2. Diversity, equity, and inclusion leadership: Nearly all institutions have diversity committees and leadership positions in this area—a great opportunity if this is an area of passion.
3. Wellness leadership: Many institutions are developing programs to support academic clinician wellness. This can include stress reduction, burnout prevention, wellness, mindfulness, self-care, and other related constructs.
4. Promotion committees and processes: All institutions also have opportunities for leadership as the head of an individual's promotion committees, or taking on a role in the institution's promotion process.
5. Interim positions: There are times where leadership roles are vacant. Someone retires and there is a gap before a new leader joins. You could consider whether being an interim

leader (of any sort) is something you might like. Very often you do not know if you would like a leadership position. It needs a lot of investigation. This is a great way to see, for yourself, if you like one type of leadership (or another). There is an end date. That can be a good thing!

What Kind of Leader Do you Want to Be?

There are many ways that you can be a leader. You can rock your own work. You can lead your own research team. That in and of itself is meritorious and entirely worthwhile. There are others, however, who want to lead not just projects but people and programs. If that is you, you have a broad list of leadership positions into which you can grow. These positions may be available in your own institution. Look for them and then look at yourself. Identify your best skills and see if they fit within these positions. They will not dilute your effect but spread your reach.

Meaningful Moments
As a faculty member, you have the opportunity to serve (literally) as a leader. Your efforts and contributions will inspire your team, promote your mission and vision, improve morale and the work environment, and enhance the quality of care your team will be able to provide. Remember that your team will look up to you as a role model, so "walk the talk" and "walk the walk" each day. Reduce the risk of burnout by aiming for a work-life balance, and adopting healthy habits for rest, sleep, diet, and exercise. Reach out to other team leaders with comparable positions to develop a consultation and support network that can provide helpful advice and support in challenging situations. You have the opportunity as a leader to make a difference for your team and your clients. Embrace it and enjoy it.
 — Yolanda (Linda) Reid-Chassiokas, MD

Being a Leader Means Building More Teams around you

In this book we have applied the SEM, mostly focusing on building a network and community around you to help you rock your science. As you navigate into roles such as mentor or leader, you become a part of other scientists' SEMs. You may be in the innermost circle as a mentor to junior scientists, and in the institutional circle for a group of faculty if you serve as a research director or division chief. Your own SEM becomes more complicated as well, as you may have more than one team in your innermost circle, or you may end up with your SEM morphing into a Venn diagram.

When you are considering taking on new roles in your institution, it is a good time to revisit your SEM (Chap. 1), your mission (Chap. 2), and your innermost circle (Chap. 3). If the new position feels like a good fit for your SEM is consistent with your goals and mission, it is time to think about who you will need on your team in this new role.

If you are taking on a research director role, you may want to meet with some other research directors to get their insights into strategies for success. You can even use the process outlined in Chap. 3 for finding mentors to identify people who may be a good fit. You may reach out to faculty from other departments, or institutions to diversify the perspectives you achieve. You may want to talk with other types of leaders, such as division chiefs or training directors, to get different perspectives on what makes a good leader. This new team can become your leadership mentoring team, who you can turn to for input and insights in your new role.

Take-Home Points
There are many leadership roles within an institution. They are framed around skills that can be developed from your own independent research career.

Lead your own work and science well. Know who is leading you at your own institution. Consider if you want to lead others too. If so, start building skills and experiences now.

Homework
- Think about your qualities that reach beyond executing research projects with fidelity and rigor.
- Identify your skills and areas of interest for present or future leadership.
- Set up some meetings with people in their positions:
  - Ask about the challenges and benefits of their role.
  - If you are intrigued by what you hear, ask for their input on what you can do now to build your experiences in that direction.
- Consider if expanding your career by overseeing others will enrich your own and help other women rock their science.

Chapter 9
Advancing in the Larger Scope of Your Field and Community

This chapter focuses on the next stages of what you can do in your professional societies. It is built on the foundation from Chap. 5, in which we discussed benefits and avenues to get involved in your professional societies and ways to stretch your skillsets as a manuscript and grant reviewer. This chapter will talk about next steps—ways to further your involvement, seek leadership roles, and expand the groups with which you interact to include organizations such as federal agencies.

Leadership: Getting Ready

Much of this chapter centers on developing paths and opportunities to leadership roles in this outer circle of your SEM. This may involve honing your leadership skills and identifying how those can be applied outside of your own research team and institution—places where people already know you well. In considering these paths and opportunities, you need to consider where your skillset in leadership is at present. This comes from self-reflection and from conversations with leaders who know you well and have seen your work over time. This process may include input from your innermost SEM circle, such as your mentors. This pro-

© The Author(s), under exclusive license to Springer Nature Switzerland AG 2024
M. A. Moreno, R. Katzenellenbogen, *Women Rock Science*,
https://doi.org/10.1007/978-3-031-48418-6_9

cess also benefits from input from your institutional SEM circle, including your division chief, center director, or research director. Those leaders may be in a good position to provide you objective feedback on your leadership style or skills, and strategies to achieve your goals.

How do you approach these discussions without feeling awkward? The set-up is important. This is not the time to "pop in" their office or catch them in the hallway. Let the discussion have an even pace. Consider starting with an email outlining your ask or your interests, alongside your rationale or related experiences. For example, explain that you are interested in advancing your career into more areas of leadership and would like feedback on your areas of strength as well as areas you could improve. Just like meeting with your mentors and bosses about your direct work and strategies for success in research, this is another ask about strategies for success in your broader career. You are asking them to comment about your skillset and not to brainstorm for job opportunities. After this written request, ask for a meeting to follow-up and get their feedback. That gives them time to reflect and does not put them on the spot to answer in that moment.

Beyond feedback on your current leadership skills, some institutions and universities offer opportunities in leadership training. These may include *classes or programs* to develop and advance leaders. One benefit of these programs is that not only do you learn key leadership skills but you gain a cohort, a peer group of like-minded future leaders who are learning alongside you. Additionally, the cost of classes or programs can be reasonable, and as such your division or department may be happy to cover the cost. In doing so, they will gain your newly minted skills, and it also reflects well on them to have members of their faculty in these programs. Before paying for these yourself, approach your mentors and leaders to inquire about support.

Another avenue to improve your leadership skills or understanding is to work more individually with a *leadership coach, sometimes called an executive coach*. This person can help you in some guided assessments of your skills or knowledge and provide resources in identified areas. Chap. 3 describes additional information about working with a coach, and Chap. 7 notes how a coach can help you hone your skills as a team leader.

And finally, you can consider pursuing *self-study* in areas of leadership. There are numerous books and courses on this topic, so being thoughtful about what you want to learn is important. The resources section at the back of this book notes a few of our favorites, you can also ask the leaders in your SEM circles for their favorite resources. You do not want to get overwhelmed or lost in an avalanche of information.

Meaningful Moments
Pediatricians are, in a large part, educators; and my interests in educating families about health and wellness soon grew beyond the classroom and exam room encounters of my day-to-day practice, Honorably discharged from the Navy, I joined the Office of Disease Prevention and Health Promotion at the Department of Health and Human Services in Washington, DC, as the Project Director of the Preventive Services Initiative. One of my duties was to work with professional organizations and universities and to educate health professionals and the public about the Healthy People Objectives and the findings of the US Preventive Services Task Force. I was also hired by the CBS station in Washington to provide medical education via health reports on the evening Eyewitness News. My tasks were supported by materials and resources provided not only by DHHS, but by professional organizations such as the American Medical Association, the American Academy of Family Physicians, and, especially, the American Academy of Pediatrics.
— Yolanda (Linda) Reid-Chassiokas, MD

Your Professional Society

Let's assume for the moment that, at this point in your career, you have been involved in your professional society for some number of years. Perhaps you have attended conferences, sat in on committee meetings, perhaps even been part of a formal committee within the society. These are the roles we discussed at the start of work within a professional society in Chap. 5.

With this work already in place, the next step to consider is whether you would like to do more in a professional society (Fig. 9.1). First, determine what roles and opportunities are available to you. While every professional society has different committees, there are a few general types of roles and committees to be aware of.

Executive Committee The executive committee is usually a smaller leadership group within the larger committee. Members of the executive committee usually have a specific period of service on the executive committee such as a three-year term. Members of the executive committee may be voted in by the larger committee or chosen by leadership. The role of the executive committee is to develop the scope and

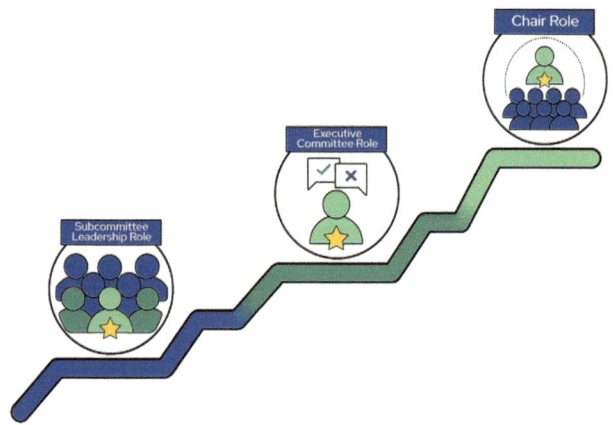

FIGURE 9.1 Leadership progression in a national committee

mission of a professional society and to assure that structure is in place for the society to complete that work.

Being involved in this type, and at this level, of a committee has several benefits to you. This includes learning more about leadership teams. You get to understand how decisions are made within the committee and how a committee is run specific to your area of science. You also get insights into larger issues within your scientific community and are a part of solving problems at this higher level. Third, you will also benefit from connections to other leaders outside of your home institution and scientific leaders who are interested in advancing their greater research field specifically in this way. These connections to other leaders may open up opportunities for collaboration, such as being invited to give presentations or collaborate on grants or projects. Finally, this work in and of itself is notable. Do not forget to document this type of leadership on your CV because as a leader in your professional society, you are demonstrating contributions to your field, and your national and international recognition. This work will likely contribute to your promotion and tenure as it demonstrates your regard among your peers.

Specific Leadership Roles Another opportunity that may arise in a professional society is being in a high leadership role within a committee. For example, the chair of the membership subcommittee, or the lead of the conference program committee may be a choice for you. These roles also offer numerous learning and networking opportunities and will help you shape the cohort of your peers and the topics that will be the focus of your scientific conferences. The workload of these roles can vary, with peaks and valleys throughout the calendar year, so it is a good idea to talk to the current or previous leadership chair to fully understand the role before taking it on (Fig. 9.2).

Committee Chairs Being the chair of a committee, rather than simply a member, is often a substantial amount of work; there are no two ways about it. These roles take ongoing time and

FIGURE   9.2 Subgroup
leadership

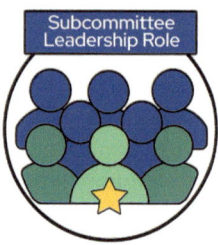

FIGURE 9.3 Committee chair

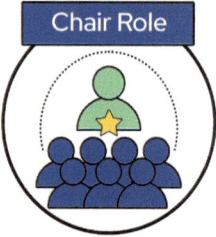

attention, and you want to be at a stage in your research that
you can take this type of work on without losing forward
movement and progress in your own work (Fig. 9.3).

As you can probably surmise, many scientists follow a progression of roles within a committee. They start out as committee members in their early career. During this time, they
identify committees that they are most interested in contributing to over the long term. By staying with and being an
active participant in a committee over time, they develop a
reputation and network within that committee. They then
may choose to run for a committee or subcommittee leadership role, then for an executive committee role, and finally for
a chair role. This progression, albeit logical, is not always
guaranteed or desirable for each individual; however, this is
often the way that leadership is grown in professional society
committees.

Journal Involvement: Beyond Reviews

In Chap. 5, we described benefits of getting involved in reviewing manuscripts for journals. This work can contribute to your knowledge of new findings in your field, as well as helping you become a better writer. In this section we would like to discuss getting more involved in journals.

As you progress in your field of work and publish more papers, you will only get more invitations to review journal articles. Thus, you should determine how and when to say yes or no to these increasing requests for reviews. Each person's decision process is unique in this area, but you will want to have your own process to guide your decisions. Here are things to consider.

1. Some scientists set limits on the number of reviews they will do each month. After a set number of reviews are completed for that month, they decline any further invitations.
2. Some scientists focus their reviews on 1–2 journals that they are very invested in and always say "yes" to those reviews. This is a good strategy if you are interested in the potential of an Editorial Board membership in the future, as you will be building a relationship with a journal and providing consistent insightful reviews when asked.
3. Some scientists choose to involve junior colleagues or mentees in reviews, allowing them to build their skills in doing the review alongside you.
4. Some scientists want exposure to as many journals and approaches as possible, so they accept reviewer invitations from new journals as priority over repeat requests. This allows your name to get out across different journals and in different areas of work.
5. Some scientists do reviews only during months in which there are not major deadlines and events. For example, if your professional society meeting is in March, and you have a grant deadline in April, you may choose to decline any invitations in those months.
6. Some scientists do reviews only of certain topic areas, keeping their scope of work narrow.

Editorial Board Positions Every scientific journal has an Editorial Board, and responsibilities of those board members may vary. In many cases, the Editorial Board does not receive any stipend (beyond experience and prestige) for this work. Some of the common Editorial Board opportunities and responsibilities may include:

1. Preferential submission of your own work to that journal (though it is unclear whether this is ever really monitored).
2. Attending a yearly Editorial Board meeting. This meeting may take place at your professional society meeting or may be distinct from it depending on whether the journal is published as a part of the professional society.
3. Participating in pre-review of certain manuscripts. The Editor may send an Editorial Board member a manuscript for a pre-review to determine if you think the paper merits being sent out for review. The benefit to the journal is to have on-hand these experts to do quick perusals of papers and deciding which are worth sending out for review, thus reducing the workload on the reviewers.

The workload involved in being on an Editorial Board may vary, but certain principles apply. You need to be ready to contribute in a timely manner when asked, so you must be in a professional position where you can fit in these unscheduled asks by your journal. You need to be able to quickly assess and confidently describe your impressions and feedback (Fig. 9.4).

FIGURE 9.4 Group membership

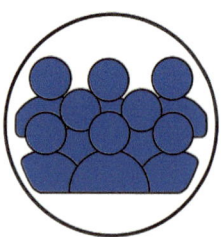

The benefits of being involved as an Editorial Board member are many. Like being in a leadership position within a professional society, as an editorial board member you have another opportunity to contribute to your field of science on a grander scale. You can help decide on what a journal's priorities might be for the coming year or whether a study merits being sent out for review. You can leverage your training and experience to help with these big and important decisions. You can also learn a lot about how scientific publishing works, develop connections to other leaders that you can learn much from, and become a bit more immersed in your own field.

Associate Editors and Editor-in-Chief Every scientific journal also has Associate Editors, who are charged with initial review of papers. This initial review leads to a decision of whether to send the paper to reviewers, and a selection and invitation of those reviewers. Thus, associate editors have a more involved role than the Editorial Board, as they oversee the daily operations of a journal. Typically, these positions are paid or have a yearly stipend. This is a much heavier level of involvement and a great way to contribute involvement to shaping the field of work beyond your research focus. However, because it is a role that involves significant investment of time on a consistent basis, it is important to balance this different type of work and responsibility with your ongoing research mission to ensure it is a good fit.

Finally, every journal has an Editor-In-Chief. This is a very prestigious position, with decision-making power and decision-making stressors that come with it. This type of position cannot help but put a damper on your own personal scientific output, but it can also open many doors to influencing the field of science as a whole.

Grant Review

In Chap. 5, we outlined ways to consider engaging in grant review opportunities early in your career. The benefits of grant review include developing insights into how to write compelling grants that can greatly improve your own grant writing. These grant reviews can be on local review groups, or even as a temporary study section (scientific review group) member for NIH. In this chapter we will discuss taking the next steps in grant reviews, such as reviewing for the NIH as a regular study section member or other federal agencies (Fig. 9.5).

How do you know if you are ready to review grants at the federal level? A first checkpoint is, as always, whether you are up to date and in a stable place with your own work. The criteria for NIH are quite specific. The Center for Scientific Review states you need to have: a current, active funding from NIH that is a R01 or equivalent; an active research program; understand the process of review; and will review applications with integrity. Diversity is also important to NIH and as such, the CSR wants members from a diversity of backgrounds. So, NIH wants grants to be reviewed by peers and by people who evaluate the science from a common, yet diverse, background and understanding.

Being involved in ongoing federal grant review often involves making a multiyear commitment. Study sections at NIH meet three times a year to review grants, and the standard commitment of membership is for 4 years, assuring a 25% turnover of members every year. If you are struggling with your own funding, or considering changing institutions, these are not the right times to take on a multiyear review

FIGURE 9.5 Grant reviewer

committee membership. Ideally, like NIH stipulates, providing reviews in these arenas would begin at the time point in which you have established a track record of publications in your area of science, and success as an investigator in getting your own federal funding.

Meaningful Moments

My advice is to build an area of expertise that you can offer in a peer review environment, have a public face in that area by publishing or other means of dissemination of information, and by all means reach out to scientific review officers and ask what they require. Be open to all possible tasks that could be step towards your participation in a community of science. Guaranteed you will learn more from the experiences than you will input, and the collaboration and learning will be invaluable in forming your own contributions.

—Marsha Lopez, PhD

There are opportunities to serve as a reviewer for grants across several federal grant institutions, including the National Institutes of Health (NIH), the National Institute of Justice (NIJ), and the National Science Foundation (NSF). These opportunities may include doing *ad hoc review* or being on a *standing review committee*.

Ad hoc reviews means you are joining the review committee for a single session. You are a temporary member. You may be invited to do an ad hoc review for a specific grant opportunity, or Research Funding Announcement (RFA) that is related to your type of research. In this case, all members of that review committee are ad hoc for that particular RFA. You may also be invited by a scientific review officer to attend one meeting of a standing review committee. This may be because that committee received applications in your area of expertise, and they feel that based on your research focus and standing in the field you would be a valuable contributor at that review session.

Being on a *standing review committee* is usually by invitation of the committee chairperson and the scientific review officer assigned to that study section. Review committees are carefully chosen to balance scientific expertise, as well as demographic characteristics of members, including geographic representation. As noted above, committee members usually serve a certain time length on the committee and are expected to attend review meetings on a regular basis. It is considered an honor and a professional milestone to join a standing review committee. It provides you with another professional home in your review committee, as you will be working together and seeing each other in person on a regular basis for years. You will have ongoing opportunities to learn about grant writing, grant review, and how review and funding decisions are made at the higher levels. This is truly learning by doing through committing to service within your scientific field. You are provided a small stipend for your work doing reviews, but it is definitely not enough to cover the time, investment, and work you are doing. So it is not worth doing for the money, but it is a nice recognition of your work.

Community Involvement

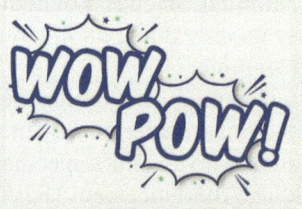

As a junior faculty, Camila developed a collaboration with Centro Hispano in her community. Her research focused on cervical cancer screening rates among Latina women, and she developed an Advisory Board of women from the center to help her design projects and translate findings to the community. A few years later, soon after achieving Associate Professor, Centro approached her to ask if she was interested in advising them on a new outreach effort. They offered to provide her 10% salary support for the next 2 years to dedicate time to this work, and to take the role of academic lead and work with an assigned community lead. This new role provided Camila support for her time, and a new leadership opportunity. Camila discussed this opportunity with her mentor and promotion committee, and they provided strong support. Camila was thrilled to accept this position.

Community involvement provides many ways to expand the impact of your science in tangible ways. In Chap. 5, we outlined ways to reach out to community organizations with relevance to your area of science, both through encouraging or inspiring the next generation of scientists and through connecting to organizations that have relevance in your own work. Examples included being part of youth-focused programs to encourage science careers, or connecting to a local LGBTQI+ organization if your work includes related health topics (Fig. 9.6).

If you have these community connections, now may be a time to advance as a leader or contributor in those organizations. One way to do this is to be part of an organization's advisory board. Like being an executive committee member or leader in a professional society, being an advisory board member means you get to guide the focus and mission of an organization that matters to you. Being part of an advisory board can bring responsibilities, such as fundraising. They

Figure 9.6 Community work

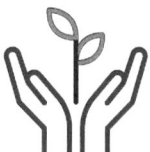

may even require directly contributing your own financial support to the organization. So these responsibilities are not usually feasible or attractive to a junior scientist. However, they can become more worthwhile and feasible at later stages in one's career and can be a way to feel direct impact on your own community. These connections can also begin to pay off in other opportunities, such as opening doors for recruitment for your studies, opportunities to give research presentations within the community, or even grassroots support for research projects that you collaboratively develop.

If you have been involved in your community and noted a gap in availability of a type of program you want to be involved in, now can also be a time to determine if this is a program you want to start yourself. For example, if you want to volunteer in a youth program to promote careers in science but you have not found one, consider starting one. You may choose to start small, with a one-day program in which youth come and get exposure to different careers in science, with simple didactics about how to prepare for a career in science. You may expand to starting a summer program for youth, shadowing researchers in their labs. If you are starting something yourself, you get to make it as big or small as you want.

This process can look remarkably like a grant application. You probably want to start by seeking other people who have similar projects and ask for their advice and insights. Then you probably want to find potential collaborators, which may include other scientists or community members such as science teachers or guidance counselors. You can then write a proposal, create a budget, and seek out funding. Your potential funders may include your own institution. In some cases, universities or research centers are hungry for opportunities to host a program such as this, as it fulfills their own community mission and also provides positive press for the institution. In some cases, funding may come from other community organizations such as the YMCA or other youth-focused organizations. There are even NIH grants, such as the R25 mechanism, that you can apply for to host your own scientific educational program.

Big One-Time Projects

Meaningful Moments

I was actively involved in drafting a resolution calling for greater "Tribal Ownership of Health-Related Data." The Resolution was unanimously passed by members of the Northwest Portland Area Indian Health Board in July 2005, and serves as a formal statement to researchers and funding agencies, calling for unequivocal tribal ownership of data collected among the Northwest Tribes. For decades, Tribes have been the subject of medical and anthropological research, with few benefits returning to the tribe as a result of their participation. In doing so, researchers have failed to recognize tribal sovereignty and their right to self-determination. Both in the Northwest and in other regions of Indian Country, concerns about tribal "ownership" have arisen upon discovery of unethical research practices. The Resolution that was passed by the NPAIHB was designed to pre-empt such occurrences in the Northwest. This Resolution gained national recognition and interest by tribes throughout North America, and was adopted in February 2006 by the National Congress of American Indians.
—Stephanie Craig Rushing, PhD, MPH

Another area of opportunity can be loosely labeled as "big one-time projects." These are opportunities to join in on a particular collaborative, join a group in writing a policy, work on a particular resolution, be part of a consensus study or join a coalition. We are calling these one-time projects, because typically you are recruited or invited to be part of the project for a designated time frame. These time frames may be quite varied, anything from being part of a one-day meeting to being in a two-year consensus study toward creation of policy recommendations. It is important to note that these big one-time projects often lead to further opportunities through the experience and connections you gain in that project. These are often fantastic career-changing opportunities that may be overlooked in your career planning.

Lessons from the Lab

Several years ago, I (Megan) was invited to be part of a big one-time project: a National Academies of Sciences Consensus Study focused on bullying. After spending some time addressing my own imposter syndrome concerns, I signed on…with some remaining trepidation. The project involved being in a coalition whose task included reviewing all of the salient literature about bullying (yes, all of it). We synthesized this existing evidence to develop a summary report, and to formulate consensus-driven policy recommendations. The work involved travel to several in-person meetings, countless hours reading and writing, and a lot of time in discussion with the coalition members and National Academies' staff both in person and via email. The end of the project, and the release of the report, brought feelings of relief and some sadness that it was all over. In reflection, this big one-time project gave me so much. I developed new connections to other researchers and federal policy-makers. I gained new experiences in translating evidence to policy and practice recommendations. Last, I have enjoyed a bevy of new research ideas, as well as potential collaborators with whom I can pursue those ideas. The benefits definitely expanded beyond the one-time nature of the project.

Multicenter Trials

Another opportunity that may arise is to be part of large, multicenter trials. Below we include a story that gets at the opportunities provided by being part of a multicenter trial, as well as the importance of having mentorship to do so.

> *I was invited to participate as a clinical investigator in a multicenter, longitudinal study of a progressive eye disease. I had recently transitioned from clinical practice to a full-time faculty appointment at a fledgling optometry program. As a faculty member from my alma mater introduced our team to the study protocol, I was apprehensive about my new responsibilities. In response to my concern, this individual, who would become an influential career-long mentor to me, provided not only direction to accomplish the immediate task—a memorable instruction to follow the "effing" protocol—but also opportunities for publication and future professional growth.*
>
> *My participation in the project led to other collaborative research as well as to more active participation in a professional organization and a working relationship with our research study chairperson who continues to this day to be a strong female mentor to me. Throughout this research project, I was also fortunate to learn from an experienced faculty member at my own institution who provided sound guidance and a sense of humor as he mentored me in classroom teaching and directed me through the idiosyncrasies of academia and a new program.*
>
> *Fast forward to the present: I completed 20+ years of service before returning to my alma mater where I now report to my former study chairperson. As I return home from a weekend away with colleagues—now friends—from across the country, I am reminded of the warmth and cohesiveness of my professional community. I am thankful for the numerous mentors that have contributed to multidimensional aspects of my professional growth.*
>
> *—Heidi Wagner, OD*

Take-Home Points

As a researcher, you can grow as a leader in professional societies, journals, funding agencies, and community groups.

Decide if being a leader in these outer circles of your SEM adds to your work as a researcher and expands your career.

Homework

- Write out your goals for advancement in your professional societies and strategies for achieving these goals.
- Write out your goals for next steps in journal and grant reviewing and strategies for achieving these goals.
- Consider your preferred ways of being involved in your community and how you see advancement in that area.
  - Brainstorm strategies for achieving those goals, including relationships or collaborators you want to seek out early.

Chapter 10
Your Forever Skills: An Epilogue

We will begin as we started. If you are woman or non-binary person in clinically relevant science, we wrote this book for you. If you are reading this book and belong to another gender category, we are thrilled that you joined us. We wrote this book with a specific framework in mind, the socioecological framework. We did this to place emphasis on you, as a scientist, in your own context. Just as your independent research fits in a larger framework of science, you as a scientist are part of a larger community of scientists. We hope that you have learned new ways to navigate, utilize, explore, and leverage your own socioecological model. We hope you have gained confidence and skills in seeking mentors, finding your professional home, and planning for your promotion (Fig. 10.1).

We are acutely aware that doing research requires more than just building a support structure for yourself. It requires numerous scientific skillsets and deep levels of knowledge. For yourself:

> You need to understand the scientific process and to know of the existing foundational data in your area of work.
> You need to know how to ask research questions and plan methodologically sound studies to address those questions.
> You need skillsets in data analysis and interpretation.

M. A. Moreno, R. Katzenellenbogen, *Women Rock Science*, https://doi.org/10.1007/978-3-031-48418-6_10

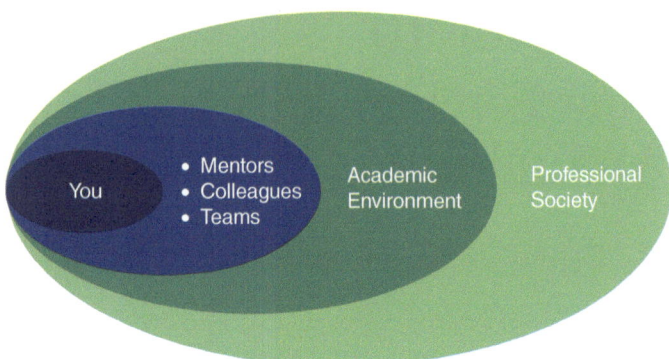

FIGURE 10.1 The socioecological model

You need to know how to communicate your findings to the world through writing and speaking.

Furthermore, as a scientist there are other skills that you will need to rock your science. These are ones that help you work as a team, lead a complex group, disseminate your work, advocate for change, and advance your field. For your team:

You need a set of management skills to run your research lab (Fig. 10.2).
You need the confidence to seek scientific collaboration that will enhance your work (Fig. 10.3).

FIGURE 10.2 CEO

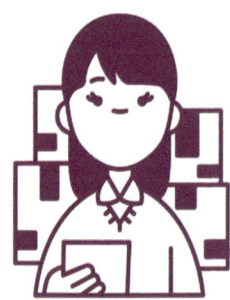

FIGURE   10.3 Scientific collaborations

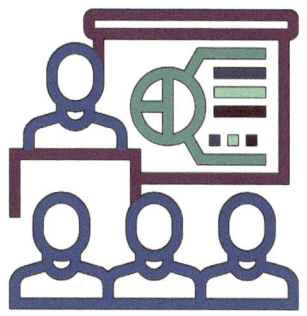

We touch on all of these skills in this book. However, this book does not provide in-depth information about each of these skillsets, and we would be remiss if we did not mention their importance. There are many other resources to seek for these critical skills and data. If you are at a loss for resources, do not forget your SEM. Use it. Ask your mentors, advisors, role models, and near-peer mentors for help. Use your institution to identify new sources of training. See if your professional society provides these learning opportunities.

As a scientist and researcher, you know that your field is constantly evolving. New data. New techniques. New methods of study design. The same will be true within and throughout your career. You will always be in a place where your own continuing education is important. Do not forget that. Think about the newest skills you want to learn, or older skills you want to master, whether they are hard skills or soft skills. And do not forget that you love to learn—that is what science is all about. Answering the unknown is your calling. Use that energy to advance your own career, your own science, and the careers of the people on your team.

Meaningful Moments
Climbing initiates the faculty process through with you make critical decisions about career development and use creativity to advance new knowledge...climbing, however, is tremendous work because while there are periods of ease...it is for the most part uphill. You have to stay focused and productive when time appears to be your own, remain confident and committed when your momentum slows.
—Maria Trent, MD, MPH

Our focus on the areas addressed in this book was selective and mindful. Growing evidence illustrates that women's strengths in leadership often include building networks and empowering others. Our book honors these strengths by addressing ways to build those networks and grow as a scientific leader and mentor. Additionally, as scientists ourselves, we are acutely aware that women, trans-, and non-binary scientists continue to drop out of the fields of science and academic medicine for various reasons. From what we have seen and what evidence exists, these reasons do not include a lack of scientific knowledge or skills. We have noted that some of these scientists who leave the field have struggled with a faulty support structure, lack of mentoring, or challenges to their confidence. We hope that books like ours will place emphasis on building one's own socioecological model and feeling confident in one's place in the scientific world. We hope books like ours will give you the confidence to begin building your own SEM, defining your own mission, and not just doing...but rocking your science.

Be part of a larger community of women and gender diverse scientists.

Share your triumphs and challenges.

Offer new ideas for how other people can build their SEM and rock their science.

Thank you for spending some time with us and we hope you will feel free to keep in touch.

References

A Few Favorite Resources

Academic Science

1. Laura Bonetta (Editor). Making the Right Moves: A Practical Guide to Scientific Management for Postdocs and New Faculty: Second Edition. Burroughs Wellcome Fund and Howard Hughes Medical Institute, USA. (2006).
2. Jeremy Boss and Susan Eckert. Academic Scientists at Work. (Second Edition). Springer Science + Business Media, LLC, New York, NY, USA. (2006). ISBN: 0-387-32176-4
3. Stephanie A. Fryberg and Ernesto Javier Martinez. The Truly Diverse Faculty: New Dialogues in American Higher Education. Palgrave Macmillan, St. Martin's Press LLC, New York, NY, USA. (2014). ISBN: 978-1-137-45605-2
4. Athene Donald (blog). www.occamstypewriter.org/athenedonald. Twitter @AtheneDonald

Jobs and Promotion

5. Victor A. Bloomfield and Esam E. El-Fakahany. The Chicago guide to your career in science. Chicago Guides to Academic Life, University of Chicago Press, Chicago, IL, USA. (2008). ISBN: 9780226060644

© The Editor(s) (if applicable) and The Author(s), under exclusive license to Springer Nature Switzerland AG 2024
M. A. Moreno, R. Katzenellenbogen, *Women Rock Science*,
https://doi.org/10.1007/978-3-031-48418-6

6. Julia Miller Vick, Jennifer S. Furlong and Roseanne Lurie. The Academic Job Search Handbook: Fifth Edition. University of Pennsylvania Press, Philadelphia, Pennsylvania, USA. (2016). ISBN: 0812223403
7. Robert M. Diamond. Preparing for Promotion, Tenure and Annual Review: A faculty Guide: Second Edition. Anker Publishing Company, Inc., Bolton, Massachusetts, USA. (2004). ISBN: 1-882982-72-X

Your Team and Mentorship

8. Sambunjak D, Straus SE, Marušić A. Mentoring in Academic Medicine: A Systematic Review. JAMA. 2006:296(9): 1103-1115. doi:https://doi.org/10.1001/jama.296.9.1103
9. Pololi L, Knight S. Mentoring Faculty in Academic Medicine: A New Paradigm? J Gen Int Med. 2005;20(9):866-870. doi: https://doi.org/10.1111/j.1525-1497.2005.05007.x
10. Goldberg, MA, Kaiser, UB. Editorial: The Rise of the Asterisk: One Step to Facilitate Team Science. Mol Endocrinol. 2015 June 29 (7): 943-5. doi: https://doi.org/10.1210/me.2015-1140
11. William R Miller and Stephen Rollnick (Editors). Motivational interviewing: Helping People Change: Third Edition. The Guildford Press, New York, NY, USA. (2013). ISBN: 1609182278

Developing New Research Ideas

12. Creative Confidence by David Kelley and Tom Kelley. Crown Publishing Group, Random House Company, New York (2013). ISBN: 978-0-385-34936-9
13. Stuart Firestein. Failure: Why Science is so successful. Oxford University Press (2015). ISBN: 019939010X

Grants and Funding

14. Jacobson RM, Fairbrother G, Sheldrick RC, Szilagyi PG. The Role of the Peer Reviewer. Academic Pediatrics. March 2017 Volume 17, Issue 2, 105-106. doi: https://doi.org/10.1016/j.acap.2016.08.011

15. On Being a Scientist: A Guide to Responsible Conduct in Research: Third Edition (2009). Published by the National Academy of Sciences: National Academy of Engineering; Institute of Medicine; Committee on Science, Engineering and Public Policy. The National Academies Press, Washington, D.C. USA. ISBN: 0-309-11970-7
16. NIH Websites for grants and review information: https://grants.nih.gov/grants/policy/review.htm; https://public.csr.nih.gov/ReviewerResources/BecomeAReviewer/ECR/Pages/default.aspx; https://public.csr.nih.gov/ReviewerResources/BecomeAReviewer/Pages/default.aspx; https://public.csr.nih.gov/ReviewerResources/BecomeAReviewer/Pages/How-Scientists-Are-Selected.aspx; Mock grant review video on the NIH website or YouTube

Writing

17. Paul J Silvia. How to Write a Lot. American Psychological Association. Washington, DC. ISBN: 1591477433.
18. Duke Graduate School Scientific Writing Resource. https://sites.duke.edu/scientificwriting/

Time Management

19. John Adair and Melanie Allen. Time management and personal development. Thorogood Publishing, Inc. London, UK. (2003). ISBN: 1-85418-223-4
20. David Allen. Getting Things Done: The Art of Stress-Free Productivity. Penguin Books, New York, NY, USA. (2015). ISBN: 0-14-20.0028-0
21. Atul Gawande. The Checklist Manifesto: How to get things right. Metropolitan Books, Henry Holt and Company, New York, NY (2009). ISBN: 978-0-8050-9174-8
22. Jocely Glei (Editor). Manage your day-to-day: Build your routine, find your focus & sharpen your creative mind. Amazon Publishing, Las Vegas, NV, USA. (2013). ISBN: 1477800670
23. Stephen R Covey. The 7 Habits of Highly Effective People. Simon & Schuster, New York, NY, USA. (1989, 2004). ISBN: 978-1-4516-3961-2

24. Project Management Website: www.basecamp.org
25. Organizing your to-dos and life: Bullet Journal: www.bulletjour-nal.com

Leadership and Communication Skills

26. Eagly A, Carli LL. Women and the Labyrinth of Leadership. Harvard Business Review. Sept 2007.
27. Sally Helgeson. The Female Advantage: Women's Ways of Leadership. Doubleday, New York, NY, USA. (1995). ISBN: 0-385-41911-2
28. Daniel Goleman. Working with Emotional Intelligence. Bantam Dell, New York, NY, USA. (1998) ISBN: 0-553-37858-9
29. Jim Collins. Good to Great. HarperCollins, New York, NY, USA. (2001). ISBN: 0-06-662-99-6
30. Joseph Grenny, Kerry Patterson, Ron McMillan, Al Switzler, Emily Gregory. Crucial Conversations. 3rd edition. McGraw Hill. New York. (2002). ISBN: 978-1-260-47418-3.
31. Susan Scott. Fierce Conversations: Achieving success at work and in life, one conversation at a time. New American Library. New York. (2017). ISBN 9780425193372.
32. Harvard Business Review (subscription), we highly recommend signing up for the HBR "Management Tip of the Day" in your email

Work–life Balance and Well-being

33. Kelly Ward and Lisa Wolf-Wendel. Academic Motherhood: How faculty manage work and family. Rutgers University Press, New Brunswick, NJ, USA. (2012). ISBN: 978-0-8135-5385-6
34. Working Equal: Collaboration Among Academic Couples (RoutledgeFalmer Studies in Higher Education): First Edition. Edited by Elizabeth Creamer. Routledge, New York, NY, USA. (2001). ISBN: 0-8155-3545-8
35. Sarah Webber, Jessica Babal and Megan Moreno (eds). Understanding and Cultivating Well-being for the Pediatrician. Springer Nature, Switzerland. (2022). ISBN 978-3-031-10842-6.

When You Need a Laugh or a (Virtual) Community

36. Shit Academics Say: www.sasconfidential.com. Follow on various social media platforms as well.
37. For MDs: KevenMD.com (blog)
38. For PhDs: Fiona Whelan (blog). Beyond the Doctorate. www.beyondthedoctorate.blogspot.com. Also on social media @ FionaEWhelan

Index

© The Editor(s) (if applicable) and The Author(s), under
exclusive license to Springer Nature Switzerland AG 2024
M. A. Moreno, R. Katzenellenbogen, *Women Rock Science*,
https://doi.org/10.1007/978-3-031-48418-6